The Juice Lady's

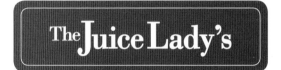

SIPPING
SKINNY

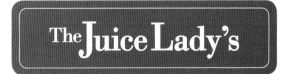

SIPPING
SKINNY

Cherie Calbom, MS

SILOAM

Most CHARISMA HOUSE BOOK GROUP products are available at special quantity discounts for bulk purchase for sales promotions, premiums, fund-raising, and educational needs. For details, write Charisma House Book Group, 600 Rinehart Road, Lake Mary, Florida 32746, or telephone (407) 333-0600.

SIPPING SKINNY by Cherie Calbom, MS
Published by Siloam
Charisma Media/Charisma House Book Group
600 Rinehart Road
Lake Mary, Florida 32746
www.charismamedia.com

Cover design by Lisa Rae McClure
Design Director: Justin Evans

Visit the author's website at www.juiceladycherie.com.

Library of Congress Cataloging-in-Publication Data:
An application to register this book for cataloging has been submitted to the Library of Congress.
International Standard Book Number: 978-1-62999-467-3
E-book International Standard Book Number: 978-1-62999-468-0

Neither the publisher nor the author are engaged in rendering professional advice to the individual reader. The ideas, procedures, and protocols contained in this book are solely for informational and educational purposes and should not be regarded as a substitute for professional medical treatment. The nature of your body's health condition is complex and unique. Therefore, you should consult a health professional before you begin any new exercise, nutrition, or supplementation program or if you have questions about your health. Neither the author nor the publisher shall be liable or responsible for any loss or damage allegedly arising from any information or suggestion in this book.

People and names in this book are composites of real patients created by the author from her experiences as a natural health professional. Names and details of their stories have been changed to protect their privacy, and

18 19 20 21 22 — 987654321
Printed in China

CONTENTS

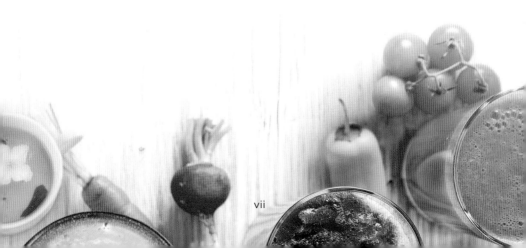

RECIPES

ACKNOWLEDGMENTS

I WANT TO EXPRESS my deep and lasting appreciation for Renae Roxanna, Taisa Efseaff Maffey, and LouAnn Hoxeng, who helped me with writing and research for this book.

A sincere thank you goes to my editor, Debbie Marrie.

Much thanks to my agent, Pamela Harty, for her help, guidance, and listening ear. How blessed I have been.

Finally, my deep gratitude and continued appreciation to my husband and official sipping tester, Fr. John, and to my heavenly Father, who has always guided my life and healed my body and soul.

INTRODUCTION

H AVE YOU TRIED just about every diet known to man (or woman)? If you've worked with all sorts of plans and nothing has been successful, hold your chin up. You need look no further. I want you to succeed not just in losing weight but in gaining health. *Sipping Skinny* isn't just about melting away fat; it's about getting to the root of why you gained weight or why you have trouble losing weight.

If you have hit roadblocks, chapter 6, "When Weight Loss Plateaus Happen to Good People," is for you. I want you to have tools that can take you through life without bouncing from one diet to another. I want you to have a lifestyle you can count on to keep you trim and healthy. That's why I have included a chapter on exercise, a "Sipping Skinny Exercise Plan," and a chapter on the importance of water. I also have a chapter on metabolism boosters so you can choose foods that really do help you sip away the pounds.

Here's a quick tip: include watercress in something you sip during each day. It truly does take away the appetite. I've discovered this firsthand, and so has my husband. In fact, he just said today that when he blends the watercress soup, he doesn't feel hungry at all after eating just one bowl. And I have plenty of recipes that include watercress, along with a variety of other options to keep your taste buds free from boredom.

Are you ready to change your internal landscape? I know you can. In July 2017 I had fifty-five volunteers in my Watercress Soup Diet who did just that. For three weeks they sipped a watercress berry smoothie for breakfast and watercress soup for lunch and ate a low-carb dinner. They lost weight and gained a boatload of good health. Some of the ladies improved their thyroid health. Others got rid of pain; two ladies lost their plantar fasciitis. Another two ladies experienced an impressive drop in blood sugar—one from 359 to 116, and one from 200 to 141. People gained muscle mass and lost their unhappy mood. Energy increase was the number-one benefit. I have compiled the statistics from that study, and I'm excited to share them with you.

I saw 51 percent lose between four and six pounds in the first week on the diet. By week three nearly half of the participants had lost between six and nine pounds. The study was specifically aimed at women for whom no other weight loss programs have worked. (The Watercress Soup Diet is featured in my book, *Souping Is the New Juicing*, along with other souping recipes and insights that enable weight loss, internal cleansing, healing, and renewed energy.) It was also the cover story of the September 18, 2017, issue of *Woman's World* magazine.

Sylvia and Michell were both featured in the *Woman's World* article. Sylvia lost nineteen pounds in three weeks and dropped a size. She was ready to go on medication to lose weight because nothing had worked until she volunteered for the Watercress Soup Diet. Michell lost twelve pounds in the same time period and twenty-one inches. She dropped two sizes—from a 16–18 to a 12–14. Her plantar fasciitis also cleared up. This diet worked when no other diets had worked before. She said she had so much energy she felt like she could "jump to the moon."

The good thing about watercress is that it provides nutrients without a significant addition of calories. Considered the top super-food, this aquatic plant is one of the most nutrient-dense vegetables known to man. I believe this is one of the reasons many of the women who participated in my Watercress Soup Diet said they were not hungry after eating a bowl of this soup. In fact, many of them said cravings just disappeared. (See chapter 8 for watercress recipes.)

Here are the outstanding results of my Watercress Soup Weight Loss Study:

- Positive changes in skin—81 percent
  29 percent, very noticeable changes
  52 percent, noticeable changes
  19 percent, no change (NC)

- Positive changes in hair—57.9 percent
  8.8 percent, very noticeable changes
  49.1 percent, noticeable changes
  42.1 percent, NC

- Positive changes in nails—49.2 percent
  5.3 percent, very noticeable changes
  43.9 percent, noticeable changes
  50.8 percent, NC

- Positive antiaging—85.7 percent
  37.5 percent, noticeable changes
  48.2 percent, not sure
  14.3 percent, NC

- Energy level increase—93 percent
  58 percent, great increase of energy
  35 percent, increase
  7 percent, NC

- Mood elevation up—69 percent
  29 percent, could not tell
  2 percent, NC

- Increase in muscle mass—20 percent
  47 percent, no
  33 percent, not applicable

- Other health improvements—55 percent
  38 percent, not sure
  7 percent, NC

- Week one weight loss
  0–3 lbs.—26, or 47 percent of people
  4–6 lbs.—28, or 51 percent of people
  7–9 lbs.—1, or 2 percent of people

- Weeks 2–3 (total pounds lost)
  1–3 lbs.—9, or 17 percent of people
  4–5 lbs.—13, or 24 percent of people
  6–9 lbs.—27, or 48 percent of people
  10–19 lbs.—6, or 11 percent of people

- Inches lost
  1–3.5 in.—19, or 48 percent of people
  4–12 in.—19, or 48 percent of people
  13–22 in.—2, or 4 percent of people

Michell Lost Twelve Pounds and Twenty-One Inches

I could jump out of my skin I'm so excited! I'm down twelve pounds and twenty-one inches in three weeks. I've had a day and a half with no pain in my foot [plantar fasciitis is gone]. It has been almost a year of stretching, icing, wearing a boot when I get home from work and all night. My energy level is through the roof. Last night I had several friends/students over; they were of all ages, the youngest being twenty-two. She looked at me and said, "You look younger; oh my gosh, what are you doing?" I told them about the Watercress Soup Diet challenge and then fed them the soup for dinner. They LOVED it. I made a double batch for them, and it was all gone! People went back for seconds. My husband asked me one morning, "How long have you been doing this?" I told him a week. He was shocked: "You got that kind of results in just one week? Wow!" I definitely can tell the difference! I feel ten years younger! Last week I lost 7.5 total inches off my body. This week I lost an additional

10 inches off my body, equaling 17.5 inches in two weeks with the six pounds lost. I just told my husband today, "Look how long my hair is getting." It's so fantastic how my body is reacting to the Watercress Soup Diet.

MY OWN JOURNEY TO HEALTH AND FITNESS

I try never to promote anything I haven't tried and don't believe in. That's why I know that the suggestions and lifestyle plans in *Sipping Skinny* work. They can help you find better health and fitness. This plan is what I've done so many times to lose a few pounds, like after the holidays or a vacation. But it isn't just weight loss I'm after. It's health—not just good health, but super health. I want that for you as well.

I recently visited a doctor for a minor issue with my foot. As I answered the intake questions, I was so pleased to say I have nothing wrong with my body. I answered "no" to every question about ailments. I take no medications. I have no diseases. I attribute that to a healthy lifestyle that includes juicing and eating a whole foods clean diet, a positive attitude, a strong spiritual life of prayer, and learning to deal with stress in a more productive way. But enjoying great health was not always the case for me. I wasn't overweight, but I was not well for quite a few years.

My health journey began after I had been sick for a few years and just kept getting worse. In fact, I was so sick and tired I could barely drag myself to work. I would sleep almost the entire weekend. I finally quit my job. I wondered if I would ever feel normal again. I had chronic fatigue syndrome and fibromyalgia. They made me so sick I was unable to continue working.

I felt as though I had a never-ending flu. Constantly feverish with swollen glands and unending lethargy, I was also in constant pain. My body ached all over—a symptom of fibromyalgia.

I moved back to my father's home in Colorado to try to recover, but not one doctor had a recommendation for what I should do to facilitate healing. So I went to some health food stores and browsed while talking with some employees, and I read a few books. I decided that everything I had been doing—eating fast food, having granola for dinner, and not eating vegetables—was tearing down my health rather than healing my body.

I read about juicing and whole foods, and it made sense to me. I bought a juicer and designed a program I could follow. I kicked off my new program with a five-day juice fast. On the fifth day, my body expelled a tumor the size of a golf ball, with blue blood vessels attached. I was surprised and actually encouraged. I thought I'd be well in short order. But that was not to be the case. I continued juicing and ate a nearly perfect diet of live and whole foods for three months, along with juicing every day. There were ups and downs throughout. Some days I felt encouraged that I was making some progress, but other days I felt worse.

The days I took a step back were discouraging and made me wonder if health was my elusive dream. No one told me about detox reactions, which was what I was experiencing. I was obviously very toxic, and my body was cleansing away all that stuff that had made me sick. This caused the not-so-good days in the midst of the promising ones.

But one day I woke up early—around 8:00 a.m., which was early for me—without an alarm. I felt as if someone had given me a new body during the night. I had so much energy I actually wanted to go jogging! What had happened? This new sensation of health seemed to have appeared with the morning sun, but my body had been healing all along; the healing simply had not manifested until that day. What a wonderful sense of being alive!

I looked and felt completely renewed. With my juicer in tow and a new lifestyle fully embraced, I returned to Southern California a few weeks later to finish writing my first book. But I called what I had done a "cure." Thinking in terms of cure rather than lifestyle, I started slipping back to my old ways of eating. My scary symptoms began to return. That alarmed me. I had experienced the glorious gift of health, and I never wanted to lose it again. That's when the realization struck that this way of eating had to be my lifestyle for the rest of my life.

Shirley's High Blood Sugar Dropped

My blood sugar went from 200 to 141 in two days and now is normal [on your Watercress Soup and Smoothie Diet]. Last week I lost two pounds, and then this week I have lost two pounds and one inch off my waist. The amazing thing, though, is the health benefits. My blood sugar is staying stable, my skin issues are clearing, and my face is firmer and more elastic. I noticed this morning that my eyelashes are thicker and more brown. I don't have very thick eyelashes, so I was grateful for this result. I have less body stiffness, more energy, and I'm sleeping better and waking up with a clearer head.

WHAT WOULD YOU LIKE TO ACHIEVE?

Weight loss? Better health? More energy? It can all be yours.

Have you been on the yo-yo dieting wheel? Rather than spinning around any longer, you can skip forward to success. The old lifestyle can be forever gone. When you finish putting into action the tips and recipes in *Sipping Skinny*, your cravings and urges that once lured you to the fridge and the snack bar should have taken a hike. Make my sipping style your way of life. Just like the ladies in my Watercress Soup Diet, you can have a happier mood and the joy of looking forward to each and every day. And think about how grateful you'll be when you have corrected some health problems like some of my ladies who got rid of pain or high blood sugar. Best of all, you'll have the best chance of preventing diseases such as diabetes and heart disease or common illnesses like colds and the flu.

This is the Skinny Sip Lifestyle! I pray you'll stick with it because feeling healthy, happy, and energetic is something you will never want to lose once you find it. As one of my ladies said, "Nothing on earth tastes as good as great health!" So no matter how alluring bad foods and drinks might be, you can choose the best. Get ready to lift your glass to a new era in your life!

CHAPTER 1

SIP IT OFF!

MARY COULDN'T LOSE weight no matter what she did. It seemed she had tried every diet on the planet. Nothing worked. She'd lose five or ten pounds. Then it would come right back on. But now she was desperate. She had a special wedding to attend in six weeks, and she needed to drop twenty pounds. How would she be able to do that? If she lost the typical two pounds a week being really strict, she'd still be short eight pounds.

I advised Mary to kick off her weight loss plan with a five-day juice fast or liquid diet. With that plan, she could lose about a pound a day, maybe more. Then if she did two days of liquid fasting each week thereafter, along with following my Sipping Skinny menu plan that included a low-carb diet the other five days, she should be able to reach her goal. It worked. Mary did lose the twenty pounds. She found the perfect dress. And she had a fabulous time with family and friends.

GET YOUR STRAWS READY!

Forget about starving yourself. Gear up for refreshing sip after sip. You're on your way to seeing a dip on the bathroom scale and your clothes fitting a little looser. Think about how great you'll feel. You know what it's like after you've lost five pounds. You walk a little faster—like you found your happy step. You look a bit younger. You feel lighter. And your clothes even seem a little newer.

But before you get started, let's address the elephant in the room, shall we? Liquid diets. They seem like they're a dime a dozen, don't they? We are always hearing about them being done in Hollywood and promoted in magazines. If you're honest, you've probably tried a few already. You might have even started reading this book somewhat dubiously, unsure how Sipping Skinny could possibly be any different than any other liquid diet you've already tried. Well, it's true that you can probably lose weight on most any liquid diet. After all, when you replace the solid food you would normally eat with juices, smoothies, shakes, soups, and broths, you're stripping your caloric intake to the bone. Plain and simple, such an extreme deficit in calories inevitably results in weight loss.

But one of the problems I see with some of the liquid diets out there is that people attempt to follow them too restrictively for far too long. And many of them don't contain the nutrients you need for good health. If you've ever attempted to drink all your meals for weeks on end, you know how boring and tortuous it gets to constantly deprive yourself of satiating, solid foods you can actually sink your teeth into. All too often, people on these more extreme liquid diets end up white-knuckling it until they eventually chuck the whole thing and go on unhealthy calorie binges to feel satisfied—to feel *normal*—again. Hence, the weight loss honeymoon is cut short, the former dieter typically ends up eating more than ever before to compensate for feeling deprived for so long, and all the weight comes right back on—and usually more. This kind of dieting is simply unsustainable. Many of us have probably proven this for ourselves at least once or twice. The fact is, a diet is only as effective as it is *doable*.

"OK, Cherie," you might be thinking, "but you told Mary to go on a liquid diet initially to lose weight. How is your way any better?" If you've read any of my previous books, visited my website, or subscribed to my e-mail newsletter, you know that I am an avid proponent of periodic, short-term juice fasts (the key words being *periodic* and *short-term*) for the purpose of cleansing the major organs through elimination, relieving the body's toxic load, correcting health issues, and, yes, jump-starting weight loss in a short amount of time. But I also take into consideration what is practical and sustainable for long-term weight loss and weight maintenance. For that reason, I instructed Mary about how to eat (yes, *eat!*) following her juice fast to continue her weight loss. And that is also why Sipping Skinny is not a liquids-only program but includes solid food as well. (You can breathe a sigh of relief now.)

There is another problem I see with most liquid dieting (or most dieting, in general): there is no clear way to transition back into regular life to provide a "new normal" or sustainable lifestyle for eating. All too often, once the diet is over and the excess weight has been lost, the former dieter returns right back to his or her previous way of eating. Well, you can guess what happens, or perhaps you've experienced it yourself: all the weight comes back. This shouldn't be surprising, considering the unhealthy eating habits that made that person overweight in the first place. In short, an effective diet must not only be doable but must also be translatable into a healthy lifestyle thereafter. After all, what good is losing weight quickly if you gain it back just as quickly once the diet is over?

Both the short-term and long-term efficacy of Sipping Skinny is really summed up in its simplicity and healthy lifestyle choices. It is founded on the most basic principles of nutrition and therefore can and should be incorporated easily into anyone's regular daily life. No, you are not required to go on an indefinite juice fast and live on herbs and water the rest of your life in order to maintain your weight loss. (You can breathe another sigh of relief now.) Sipping Skinny is not about surviving on as few liquid calories as possible; rather, this program is about *abundance*. I want you to absolutely flood your body with the nutrients it needs. I want you to nourish and fuel it with satisfying, healing, and health-promoting foods—foods that your body was designed to take in and utilize for optimum energy, cellular repair, and release of health-compromising toxins, waste, and excess fat. Sipping Skinny is all about thriving on real food, especially those foods that are known to provide the most health benefits. I'm referring to those foods found in nature that are positively brimming with essential vitamins, minerals, phytonutrients, biophotons, and enzymes. What could be more glorious and sustainable than that?

Riviera Lost Ten Pounds

I shed seven pounds during Cherie's juice and raw foods retreat, equaling four belt notches, simply by participating fully in her program. One month later, NONE of it has returned, despite the fact that I was traveling for three of the four weeks! With a little research, I easily located organic restaurants and local organic juice bars, staying on track and eating clean for the most part. Since the retreat, I've shed another three pounds, but most importantly, my health is fully restored. I have the energy and positive heart attitude I need in order to face life challenges again, exercise, and make right decisions regarding life.

THE PANIC FOR PROTEIN

And finally, there is a third problem I see with one type of liquid dieting in particular. This trend in liquid dieting is so common that it deserves its own section. Alas, I'm talking about the liquid diets that center on meal replacement shakes boasting of protein. In these diets we are instructed to replace at least one meal a day, usually with our choice of a chocolate or vanilla shake, and then eat the bare minimum for our remaining meals. These magic protein shakes are promised to fill us up, keep us satisfied for hours, and take away our desire for all the foods we would normally want to eat. In fact, you've probably noticed that many food products these days are marketed on the merit that they are loaded with protein.

While protein does help curb appetite and reduce sugar cravings, it seems the message we're being given lately is that protein is the answer for everything. *Carbs making you fat? Replace all those carbs with protein instead!* We are constantly being reminded that we need more protein in our diets for the sake of both our health and our waistlines. And many consumers have responded in kind by dutifully loading up on protein—not just by eating large amounts in whole food form at meals, but by supplementing with protein powders and snack bars on the side as well. We must be the most protein-loaded country on the planet! And yet we remain one of the unhealthiest societies and one of the most obese.

Now, don't get me wrong; I am a firm believer in the health benefits of protein and encourage consuming the necessary amounts of protein the body requires—that is, if the source of protein is healthy for you and has been grown, raised, and processed without the use of chemicals, hormones, antibiotics, or unhealthy processing methods. But unlike the creators of these "weight loss shakes" would lead you to believe, this country's collective weight problem is not due to a lack of protein. On the contrary, if you look at the diets of societies with the healthiest weights, what you will find is that they consume lots of vegetables and plant-based foods and relatively small portions of lean proteins.

What's more, many of the protein-based meal replacement shakes on the market right now are loaded with synthetic ingredients. They include artificial sweeteners (or sugar), colors, and preservatives, not to mention GMO-derivatives (genetically modified organisms) like soy protein isolate, which is often the very source of protein on which these shakes are based and is one of the main ingredients. Besides the fact that the soy-derived ingredients in many meal replacement shakes are genetically modified, they are also known to be hormone disruptors. Soy proteins, especially concentrated soy proteins, contain phytoestrogens, which mimic estrogen in the body and can lead to estrogen dominance and an increased risk of cancer in both men and women.[1] Soy is also goitrogenic, which means it interferes with the thyroid's absorption of iodine and hormone production. Quite simply, many meal replacement shakes on the market today are bad for you, despite whatever health and weight loss claims they might make. Just as they say to always read the fine print, always read the ingredient list as well!

Unlike many creators of weight loss programs, I don't believe in pushing the sale of a manufactured food product that must be purchased indefinitely as long as you want to continue losing weight. This is nothing more and nothing less than a marketing ploy and doesn't teach you a way of living. Anytime you hear that the secret to weight loss success lies in a substance that's been engineered in a laboratory—such as a proprietary powder, pill, or food that can last for weeks to months on a shelf and is saturated with preservatives—I recommend that you run the other way. Such claims must be taken with not just a grain of salt but a loaded saltshaker. The obesity epidemic we are seeing today is a relatively new phenomenon in history, as are the ever-increasing rates of type 2 diabetes, cancer, and heart disease. How then did our ancestors manage their weight and maintain their health for so long before these miracle weight loss products came along? To paraphrase Maria in *The Sound of Music*, we should start at the very beginning.

WHOLE FOODS AND THEIR DEMISE...CONVENIENCE FOODS AND THEIR ALLURE

Fundamentally, the human body was designed to function and thrive on the nutrients packaged in whole foods provided by nature. I'm talking about vegetables, fruit, nuts, seeds, legumes, whole grains, animal meat, and animal products like eggs and dairy. Up until relatively recently in world history, this is solely what was available for fuel and nourishment, and this is what people were perfectly content to live on. Again, these whole foods contain all the essential vitamins, minerals, fats, and proteins the human body requires for sustenance, good health, and maintaining a healthy weight. It's as true for us now as it was for our ancestors back through the ages. We didn't suddenly get bodies adapted for convenience food.

In these modern times, however, we have access not only to whole foods but often greater access to "food-like" products—products that may look like food, smell like food, and taste like food, but are in fact made up of numerous ingredients that have been highly processed, refined, and even engineered in a lab. This includes fast food; fried food; junk food; frozen food products; boxed or prepackaged meals, such as those that come with their own seasoning or sauce packets; bottled sauces and salad dressings; and anything made with refined sugar, high-fructose corn syrup (HFCS), and refined flour. These food-like products are strategically designed to appeal to our senses (sight, smell, taste, and texture) while still assuring the end result is a product with a shelf life that will outlive *us*.

I'm not sure if you noticed, but all those food-like products listed above have something in common: they're meant to be prepared and/or consumed quickly. In other words, convenience foods. It's no secret that many of us today live fast-paced, stressful lives. Together, the demands of work life and family life seem to suck up all of our time and energy so that when it comes time to eat, we grab whatever is quickest and easiest. We wolf down bowls of cereal in the morning with our families, we throw bags of chips and fruit snacks along with pre-packaged peanut butter and jelly sandwiches and juice boxes into our kids' lunches, and then we swing by the drive-through on our way home from work. The problem is that we've grown so accustomed to eating these highly processed foods conveniently packaged in brightly colored wrappers, boxes, and plastic containers, or that we receive in greasy bags through our car windows, that we've lost sight of what real food actually is. As famed British chef Jamie Oliver reminds us, "Real food doesn't have ingredients; real food *is* ingredients."[2]

It is also true that many of us are enamored by the infinite varieties of food-like products we see on commercials, billboards, and grocery store shelves. Even in our hectic lives—or perhaps especially in our hectic lives—we manage to keep an eye out for something to treat our taste buds, to make us feel happy or comforted, or to make us feel like we're doing something nice for ourselves. It's no surprise that so many people turn to these manufactured food products because, again, they have been strategically designed to appeal to our basic needs. The food manufacturing companies' playbook is short but effective: load up the product with refined sugar, salt, fat, or any combination of the three, and then market it to allure consumers. And it works every time. Refined sugar and flour and flavor enhancers like monosodium glutamate (MSG) are incredibly addictive, so much so that consumers overindulge in these products before they even know what's happening.

Consider for a second the times you sat on the couch, watching TV, eating broccoli floret after broccoli floret or peas from the shell by the handful. Now consider how often you've eaten a whole canister of salty potato chips, a pint of ice cream, or an entire sleeve of cream-filled chocolate cookies in one sitting. Each of these scenarios depicts binge eating, and yet the latter examples with junk food are the more plausible. Why? Those food-like products purposefully contain unnatural, addictive ingredients in order to hook you and keep you coming back for more. Hence, sales are up but health is on the decline.

So what actually happens when you introduce manufactured food products into your body? Your body begins to break them down like it would real food. It takes and uses what it can from what it recognizes but doesn't know what to do with unnatural, molecularly altered substances that provide no nutritional value or serve any function in the body. The liver works to process and eliminate such toxic material, but it can only handle so much, especially considering all the other sources of toxicity it has to contend with on a daily basis. Inevitably, the foreign nonfood substances that are not eliminated from the body become stored in fat cells in order to protect the body from them.

Over time, the liver and other major organs of elimination in the body can become overburdened by all the non-food substances they routinely have to process, and thus they become sluggish—no longer able to perform their jobs efficiently. (Think about non-alcoholic fatty liver that is on the rise.) Often, one of the first signs of distress in the body from poor diet and toxicity is fatigue. This is because the body has to work so much harder to function that it tires more easily, and it requires more sleep to try to repair itself. For some, sleep becomes disturbed because the body is so run-down, stressed, and toxic. Other common signs of dysfunction in the body from poor diet and toxicity are digestive issues, such as acid reflux, heartburn, bloating, gas, constipation, and diarrhea. Left unaddressed, poor digestion and incomplete elimination of waste and toxins will turn the body into a breeding ground for disease.

One Man's Transformation (As Told by His Wife)

After reading your book *Juicing, Fasting, and Detoxing for Life*, all of a sudden I began to look at our bodies, health, and nutrition with new eyes. I started to pay attention to symptoms my husband had that he seemed to just accept as normal. Most days when my husband came home from work, typically about 5:30, he'd turn on the TV and then fall asleep within minutes. After waking up for dinner and spending some time together, he'd again fall asleep while watching TV, usually by 9:00. He had a management job in an office setting which wasn't physically demanding or particularly stressful (by his own admission), and he didn't have to wake up until 7:00 to get ready for work, so I couldn't understand why he was so tired all the time.

I also noticed he seemed to have acid reflux and gas after dinner almost nightly and would eat antacids like

9

from harm. But once you remove the toxins, you remove the threat of harm, thus the fat no longer serves a purpose and suddenly becomes expendable. When health symptoms begin to disappear as a result of good nutrition, weight loss follows quite naturally as well.

I'd like you to take note of something in particular from the letter, however, and that is this gentleman's progression of improvement. Notice that he improved from exchanging food-like products for whole foods and juicing, but it wasn't until he went on a juice fast that he experienced a truly dramatic breakthrough. Why is that? If eating whole foods was good enough for our ancestors to receive their necessary nutrition and maintain healthy weights, then why shouldn't it be enough for us? Why should we need to supplement with juicing or resort to liquid diets from time to time?

The answer is that our ancestors were not exposed to all the toxins that we are today. From air pollution to heavy metals in our soil, water, and fish to pesticides on our produce to plastic packaging of our food to all those food-like products saturated with preservatives we've been talking about—and everything in between—the current general population on this earth is exposed to more toxicity than ever before. To be sure, eating a whole foods diet abundant in fresh, raw vegetables is the foundation we all need to receive proper nutrition, to maintain our health, and to maintain healthy weights. However, many of us have more toxicity than our bodies can efficiently purge in a timely manner on a whole foods diet alone. Especially if you're someone with health problems and/or stubborn weight to lose, consuming concentrated amounts of nutrients in fresh, raw liquid form is the difference between chronic symptoms and healing; fatigue and renewed energy; unwanted pudge and a flat belly. It was the answer for me, and I have heard countless testimonies over the years of how it has worked for others.

So why does liquid dieting with vegetables and fruit make such a difference?

For one thing, liquid dieting with fresh, raw vegetable and fruit juices, smoothies, soups, and broths along with various flavored waters exponentially increases the amount of nutrition you can give your body at a time and boosts your metabolism. When you extract the nutrient-dense liquid from vegetables and fruit in their fresh, raw state, or purée the vegetables and fruit into a liquid, you are condensing virtually all the nutrition they contain into an easily consumable, easily digestible, and highly absorbable food. So when you follow the Sipping Skinny program, you will basically be delivering all those nourishing, healing, energy-boosting vitamins, minerals, phytonutrients, biophotons, and enzymes directly into your cells. And let me tell you, your cells will love it! In fact, the more nutrient-depleted and toxic a body is, the more the body's cells will gobble up those precious nutrients and beg for more. Hippocrates could not have given better health advice when he said, "Let food be thy medicine and medicine be thy food."[3]

By the way, have you noticed how many times so far I've specified that the juices, smoothies, soups, and broths should be "fresh" or "raw"? That wasn't an accident. Maybe you've seen the bottled or boxed juices sold in grocery stores that claim to be 100 percent natural, made of 100 percent vegetables and fruit, even 100 percent organic. Often they are even refrigerated, making you feel like they are raw and fresh as can be. The problem is that processed juices—whether bottled, canned, or frozen—have lost so many nutrients, enzymes, and biophotons in their processing that they've been reduced to a laughingstock among the fresh, raw juices that still contain all their live nutrients. Even the refrigerated juices have to be pasteurized unless they go through a special process that preserves nutrients. They are usually very expensive. If you want to flush out toxins and melt off fat, those store-bought juices simply won't cut it.

Again, think *fresh* and *raw* vegetable and fruit juices, smoothies, soups, and broths. For most people, this means *homemade*, using a juicer and/or blender, and the Sipping Skinny recipes provided in this book and many of my former books. These days, there are more juice and smoothie shops than ever before, especially in big cities. They can be a great convenience, but visiting them also adds up quickly. So unless you have the extra money to spend, and in order to receive the most benefits from the Sipping Skinny program, I recommend investing the money in a good quality juicer if you don't already have one. (See chapter 4 for recommendations on choosing a juicer.) But if you're someone who already spends five dollars on your daily morning latté, you can easily swap your hyper-stimulating, acid-producing, toxin-laden coffee for a naturally energizing, alkaline-promoting, organic juice, and you'll be even Steven. In fact, I'd argue you'd be better off, all things considered.

Another reason liquid dieting with vegetables and fruit yields such superior results is it gives the digestive system the opportunity to rest. The digestive system is constantly working, breaking down food, shuttling off nutrients to where they are needed in the body, converting excess glucose to fat and fat to glucose. The digestive system constantly requires energy to continue working. When you follow a liquid diet like Sipping Skinny, your digestive system doesn't have much of a job to do. Your food has already been broken down mechanically by a juicer or blender into a bioavailable form. As you drink your juice, smoothie, broth, or soup, it quickly slides down through the digestive system, and then the nutrients get absorbed through the walls of the small intestines into the bloodstream. In as little as twenty minutes from consuming your liquid meal, all those detoxifying, life-giving nutrients are already feeding your cells. This means the energy that previously would go to your digestive system so it could do its job can now be reallocated to other parts of the body in need of repair and rejuvenation. This means detoxifying, healing, and ultimately weight loss.

The third main reason you want to choose Sipping Skinny when it comes to liquid diets is because of two letters: pH. Think back to high school chemistry class for a second. Remember that pH refers to how acidic or alkaline a substance is. The scale ranges from 0 to 14, with 7.0 being neutral. Anything above 7.0 is alkaline, while anything below 7.0 is acidic. The human body is happiest when its blood is slightly alkaline, between 7.35 and 7.45, but unfortunately many people favor eating more acid-producing foods than alkaline-forming foods. Even more unfortunate, if a person is too acidic, they are prone to inflammation and illness, resistant to healing, and find losing weight to be very difficult. You might say an acidic body has something like a death grip on fat. To put it bluntly, if you want to heal your body and/or lose excess weight, you must achieve a balanced pH by increasing alkalinity.

Sipping Skinny to the rescue! At this point, it shouldn't surprise you to learn that some of the most alkaline foods you can eat include vegetables and fruit; therefore, fresh, raw vegetable and fruit juices and smoothies as well as vegetable soups and broths are incredibly alkalizing for the body. Consuming a high-alkaline liquid diet makes weight loss easier than ever because the nutrients are so easily absorbed and quickly utilized to alkalize and energize the body on the spot. Other alkaline foods to keep in your diet include legumes like beans, lentils, and split peas, as well as nuts and seeds.

It is important to keep in mind that whether a food is acidic or alkaline is determined not by its original state but rather its state after it has been processed in the body. For example, it may surprise you to learn that dairy produces acid in the body, even though it is an alkaline substance to begin with. And remember our talk earlier about the current preoccupation with protein? Protein-rich foods like meat, fish, and eggs are also highly acidic for the body. Hopefully this gives you one more reason not to jump on the protein indulging bandwagon but to instead eat protein in moderation. It's not that you should never eat meat or eggs (I certainly do), but simply that acidic foods should not form the bulk of your daily diet. Ideally, no more than about 25 percent of your diet should be from acidic foods and the remaining 75 percent from alkaline-forming foods. This is also one more reason to shy away from convenience foods, which are notoriously acid-producing...and just plain bad for you!

The consensus among most health professionals is that certain foods produce acidity in the body whereas others produce alkalinity. You want to refer to these lists to limit or in some cases avoid acid-producing foods and increase alkaline-forming foods.

ACIDIC FOODS	ALKALINE FOODS
Alcohol (wine, beer, liquor)	Fruit
Black tea	Legumes (beans, lentils, split peas)
Coffee	Nuts and seeds
Dairy	Sprouts
Eggs	Vegetable juices
Fish	Vegetables
Grains	
Junk food	
Meat	
Oxidized oils	
Soda pop	
Sports drinks	
Sugar and sweets	
Trans fats	

Once you back away from a diet dominant in acidic foods and beverages and up your intake of vegetables and fruit—including vegetable and fruit juices, smoothies, soups, and broths—you'll notice your body doesn't hang on to fat as it did before. As you achieve a better balance of alkalinity versus acidity, the body is freed up to release excess fat. Your metabolism will also improve because an alkaline environment is ideal for adrenal and thyroid health. Too much acid in the body means slow hormone activity, which means the body won't readily convert calories and fat into energy to burn. There are many people in this condition who try to eat as minimally as possible and still can't seem to lose weight. What they don't realize is that it's not a matter of how much they're eating but rather *what* they're eating. But once they switch to an alkalizing, pH balancing, nutrient-rich diet, their hormones shift back into balance and their metabolism kicks back into gear. The bottom line—favoring an alkaline-rich diet only leads to better health, happier hormones, improved metabolism, and easier weight loss. And that's the whole point, isn't it?

YOU *CAN* GET SOME SA-TIS-FAC-TION... FROM SIPPING SKINNY!

Have you noticed that when you eat nutrient-depleted foods, like your standard junk food with all its refined sugars and carbohydrates, you don't ever really feel full or satisfied? To echo Kenny Chesney in the song, "You and Tequila," we will find that one is too many and we'll never be satisfied with one more. For most of us, one serving of chips or one scoop of ice cream is rarely enough. Or have you noticed that you may feel full immediately after a fast food or high-carb meal, but then you feel hungry again within just a few hours? (This is a phenomenon many people have experienced and joked about regarding Americanized Chinese food, which includes mostly dishes with sugary sauces and lots of white rice, which is highly refined and has been stripped of its nutrients and turns to sugar easily.) You may have eaten a large amount of food like this but your body remains unfulfilled because it needs nutrients that it's not getting. When you feed your body nutrient-depleted food, regardless of the calorie count, it can never reach full or long-lasting satisfaction. And so you eat more. And more. Again, food-like products and refined foods initially seem like they're your friends because they taste so good, but they're really your enemy. They trick you into thinking you feel good when you eat them, but they never quite satisfy, so you have to keep eating them to try to feel good again. In the end, they only make you gain weight and feel bad. They lure you down the road to death.

On the contrary, what you will notice as you "Sip Skinny" is how satisfied you are after you drink down a glass of juice or smoothie, or take in the last spoonful of a soup or broth. You might wonder how this can be true when you're consuming so few calories and it's all in liquid form. It is estimated that the nutrients in fresh, raw liquids like those in the Sipping Skinny program are at work in your system somewhere between twenty and thirty minutes. This means all those amazing nutrients are rushed into your cells in record time. This signals your brain that you've been well fed and you have the nourishment you need for the time being. Plus, when you satisfy your body with nutrient-dense juices and other healthful liquids, your blood sugar stabilizes and your appetite for junk food, sweets, and high-carb foods fades away. It's a win-win!

THE STORY OF REPLENZA

Once upon a time in the land of Plentitude lived a lovely girl named Replenza. As she grew into a young woman, she became what the locals called "the most beautiful woman in the land." With shining, long blond hair and a glowing, rosy complexion, her features and curves caught the eye of the most eligible young men of the country. Replenza was the talk of the village and far beyond. This praise caught the attention of the Queen Maddee, who had always held that title until she aged and Replenza stripped her of her fame. Her jealously of Replenza grew by the day until she could no longer sit idly in her stone castle, not far from Replenza's modest home. She devised a plan to not only remove Replenza from sight, but to destroy her beauty.

Late one summer afternoon under a blue, blue sky, while gathering vegetables and herbs from the family's garden, two palace guards approached Replenza. One of them threw an ugly gunny sack over her head, hoisted her onto the lead guard's horse, and headed for the castle tower.

Replenza was imprisoned in a room at the top.

The evil queen then set her plan into action to destroy Replenza's beauty. She made sure Replenza was fed food made mostly with sugar, refined white flour, and unhealthy cooking oils. She was given no vegetables and very few protein-rich foods. Replenza felt sicker by the day. She gained weight so quickly that her dress was bursting at the seams in no time. The queen sent unattractive large dresses for her to wear and gloated with delight.

Replenza put on a lot of water weight along with fat, because she was eating food that she was allergic to and was getting almost no activity.

In five weeks, Replenza had gained more than twenty pounds and was miserable. Three months later she was more than forty pounds overweight.

Meanwhile, strong, handsome young prince Galavant, who lived in the neighboring country and loved Replenza, was desperate to find her, as were her parents and siblings. Galavant sent scouts to look over the entire area near where she lived, but no one knew what happened to her. He would not give up. One day, one of Galavant's scouts decided to ask a young boy walking down the road with his fishing pole if he knew anything about Replenza's whereabouts. The boy's mother was one of the palace cooks—actually, the one who made Replenza's food. The lad showed Galavant's scout the tower where Replenza was imprisoned.

Since the queen was friends with Galavant's parents, the king and queen of Loveland, she did not wish to offend them, so she allowed Galavant to visit Replenza. But they could only talk through the door opening where she received her food.

Galavant was shocked when he saw the terrible state Replenza was in. He quickly devised a plan and rode home to enlist the help of his family's herbalist. He returned with recipes that included herbs, spices, vegetables, and fruit that would help Replenza lose weight. His plan was to rescue her by an escape through the tower window, but she would have to lose weight to fit through the opening. She would also need to become healthy and strong again.

Each day he brought her vegetable juices, smoothies, elixirs, teas, and soups that Replenza's mom and sisters helped to prepare according to the herbalist's instructions. The queen allowed her to have them as long as Replenza ate all her palace food. After all, she thought they would only help to make her fatter.

It was hard at first not to eat any solid food. And she had become so addicted to sugar that she had withdrawal symptoms. But she wanted to be free of her prison and to be with Galavant so much that she managed each day to scrape all her food into the gunny sack used to kidnap her. Then she hid the sack under her bed. Her room started to smell worse each day because of the spoiled food, but the guards didn't notice because they were lax in emptying her latrine buckets. Her room never smelled good. She also started a whole series of exercises to strengthen her arms and her core so she would be ready for the escape.

Replenza lost a lot of water weight quickly on her liquid diet. The ugly clothes got looser and looser, but the guards didn't notice because the clothes were large to begin with. She began to feel better each day, more like herself again. One day she decided to try on her own dress. Though a little tight, it fit.

The next day, when Galavant came with her liquid meals, Replenza whispered that she thought she could slip through the window. They devised a plan of escape. The next day, he would hide a long rope in a basket with the juices and soups. Her mom would make her famous apple pie, and Galavant would offer the guard a piece as he often had in the past. When the guard was busy eating the pie, he'd slip the rope through her door window. When night would fall, she'd tie it to the metal strip in the middle of the double window, slip out through the opening, and climb down the rope with her feet steadied against the stone-gray wall. Galavant would be there with Replenza's family to catch her if she fell. He would come in the middle of the night when everyone was sleeping.

At two in the morning the next day, Galavant threw a small stone against Replenza's window. She had not slept one minute as she lay on her bed waiting for him to arrive. With her own dress on, and feeling stronger than ever, she was ready for the escape. Though it was difficult for her to get through the window, she finally managed to climb out and grasp the rope as she walked herself down the side of the building. All her family, including her brother and several cousins, were there with Galavant. They brought large quilts they held tightly below Replenza in case she fell. The rope was about ten feet too short. So, while she made it to the end, she had to jump the final distance to the taut quilt that the whole family held.

With tears, hugs, and kisses, Replenza was safe at last. She and Galavant rode away swiftly through the night to Loveland, where the evil queen Maddee could never harm her again. Galavant asked her to marry him. With a wedding that captured the attention of the nation, they were married in the cathedral nearest the palace. And much to Queen Maddee's dismay, Replenza was now nearly an equal. One day she would be Queen of Loveland and would be known as the most beautiful queen in the entire continent.

REPLENZA'S ELIXIRS

This fairytale story has a theme. The wicked queen is alive and well in our society, making many people sick and fat with her food. But the juices, smoothies, soups, broths, teas, and elixirs in this book can set you free from captivity if you are a prisoner to their bad effects. You can escape the prison that has held you in overweight despair or ill health. Would you like to know what was in the juices, soups, elixirs, and teas that Galavant brought Replenza? Read on. They'll work for you too, and you can escape what holds you prisoner to your weight and health challenges.

FINAL THOUGHTS AS YOU GET GOING

The Sipping Skinny program is about as easy as it gets when it comes to preparing nutritious, real food sipables and foods to eat. They will facilitate your journey to better health and weight loss, but it does take more effort than opening a plastic container or cardboard box and immediately eating what's inside. Earlier I talked about how the hectic nature of our lives has reduced many of us to relying on highly processed and nutrient-depleted convenience foods to get us through the day. Unfortunately, those shortcuts come with a cost, and that cost is our health and our waistlines. Hopefully you have come to the conclusion that the sacrifice of your health and weight isn't worth it. Something has to change. You were meant to feel better, to live better. You were meant for *more*.

You would do very well to approach this book and this program as a turning point for your weight, your health, and your overall lifestyle. Sipping Skinny is about getting back to eating what your body was designed to eat, what has been provided in nature and was once unquestionable fare for our ancestors. The truth is that the solution to weight loss has been in front of us all along. We don't need to come up with something new, but rather we would all benefit by going back to the basics, back to what we used to know. The recipes for juices, smoothies, soups, and broths you will find in this book are simply the jumping-off point, waking up your body and putting it on the fast track to weight loss, but even more importantly, health and vitality. Congratulations on your decision to begin this journey! I will be cheering you on the whole way through.

CHAPTER 2

THE SKINNIEST LITTLE DRINK OF THEM ALL!

W HAT DO YOU think the healthiest zero-calorie drink is? If you said pure water, you're right. Ah, water! That clear, pure liquid we take for granted. It's right up there with eating your vegetables, which we all know is of major importance. But maybe you don't know just how important water is to your health and fitness.

A successful weight loss program is fueled by drinking a generous amount of water. If you are getting regular exercise and eating a great diet but still don't seem to be shedding those pounds, a lack of water may be the reason. Water plays a vital role in the metabolism of fat. A certain level of water is required for your kidneys to function efficiently. If they are dehydrated, the liver takes on a large amount of the workload. The liver must now divide its efforts between the kidneys' work and its own duties, which include transforming fat into energy. And it's already overworked with all the toxins in our modern world. So what does that tell you? You will lose less fat when the liver is not functioning at full capacity because it is key in metabolizing fat. Water plays a very important role in lightening its load.

FLUSH THAT FAT

Dehydration causes your metabolism to slow and thus your weight loss to slow. When you drink the recommended quantity of water on a regular basis, your metabolism stands to attention. It burns calories more efficiently and at an accelerated speed. When the body is dehydrated, fat removal slows down or stops altogether because the fat tissue does not receive proper blood flow.

According to health-care professionals, the ideal amount of water for an average person to consume in the course of a day to maintain the process crucial to weight loss is sixty-four ounces. If you are very large or significantly overweight, they recommend adding another eight ounces of water for every twenty-five pounds of extra weight.

Michael Boschmann, MD, and colleagues from Berlin's Franz-Volhard Clinical Research Center performed a study that supports this recommendation. They tracked energy expenditures among seven women and seven men who were not overweight and, for the most part, were healthy: "After drinking approximately 17 ounces of water, the subjects' metabolic rates—or the rate at which calories are burned—increased by 30 percent for both men and women. The increases occurred within 10 minutes of water consumption and reached a maximum after about 30 to 40 minutes."[1] The increase in metabolic rate between women and men also differed. In men, burning more fat fueled the increase in metabolism. In women, metabolism increased as their breakdown of carbohydrates increased.[2] Over the course of a year, the researchers estimated that a person will burn an extra 17,400 calories if they increase water intake by 1.5 liters (50.72 ounces) a day. This results in approximately five pounds of weight loss a year. So why does this happen? The body attempts to heat the ingested water, which accounts for up to 40 percent of the elevation in calorie burning.[3]

The body will go into survival mode when it doesn't have an adequate amount of water. It stores all the water it can find in preparation for an upcoming emergency. After all, there could be a drought. The body gathers it from any available area and retains it in places such as the thighs, ankles, hips, and around the stomach. Keep this in mind the next time you fly, and make sure you get plenty of water. A day of traveling can be very dehydrating, and many people complain of swollen feet and ankles by the end of the day. Before I got this message loud and clear, I had an episode where I could not get my shoes back on when we landed. I had to exit the plane barefoot with shoes in hand. Clearly, the point to remember is that one of your strongest allies in your fitness plan is water.

SIGNS OF DEHYDRATION

Mild: flushed skin, headache, fatigue, thirst, dry throat and mouth

Moderate: low blood pressure, rapid heart rate, weakness, urine that is highly concentrated (darker yellow color) but low in volume, lack of energy, and dizziness

Severe: poor circulation, muscle spasms, increased weakness, failing kidney function, and swollen tongue.

THE FOUNDATION FOR A HEALTHY AND LASTING WEIGHT LOSS

Many people believe that all liquids count as water, but this just isn't the case. It must be pure water to actually qualify as water. Often what we think is hunger is really just thirst (more on this later).

H_2O and fat burn

Your body will not perform properly without an adequate amount of water. You can last a more extensive period of time without food than you can without water. In order to proceed efficiently with its daily operations, the body requires an abundance of pure water;

weight loss depends on it. As stated earlier, the rate at which your liver burns fat increases with sufficient amounts of water, while decreasing water retention. When you are not consuming enough water, the body will hoard it.

The brain sends signals to the body that may feel like hunger but often signals the body is asking for water. When we should be drinking water, we are often eating food. This was illustrated in a study by Brigham and Women's Hospital.[4] The next time you feel hungry, grab a glass of water instead of a snack. After drinking the water, wait fifteen minutes and see if the hunger disappears.

Fereydoon Batmanghelidj, MD, (or Dr. B, as I call him), is the author of *Your Body's Many Cries for Water*. He states that people who are overweight often "don't know when they are thirsty; they don't know the difference between 'fluids and water.'"[5]

It is likely that you will eat less when you drink a glass of water twenty to thirty minutes before eating. Dr. Brenda Davy, associate professor of human nutrition, foods, and exercise at Virginia Tech, did some research that supports this claim. Her study showed that people who drank two glasses of water during this time frame before meals lost more weight initially, and in the long term, versus people who didn't. Dr. Davy and her team published another study in the *Journal of the American Dietetic Association*. They discovered that people consumed an average of seventy-five fewer calories at a meal when they drank water first. That may seem minuscule, but you could lose about 14.5 pounds in a year by just eating seventy-five fewer calories at lunch and dinner and drinking more water during the day. But here's a real eye-catcher: an interference in weight loss will occur and metabolism will drop if you are even 1 percent dehydrated.[6]

SIPPING SKINNY WATER TIPS

1. Drinking water reduces bloating.
2. Muscles perform at their peak with adequate water.
3. Drinking water promotes weight loss by preventing constipation.
4. Drinking water can elevate mood and improve brain function.
5. You may eat less and feel more satisfied when you drink water before a meal.
6. To limit snacking, grab a large glass of water instead. It will fend off cravings and fill you up, which will help you to lose weight.
7. Drinking water promotes clearer skin.
8. Drinking water can assist in the prevention and treatment of headaches.
9. Water helps the kidneys flush out toxins and cleanses the entire body.

WATER SIPPING IN SCHOOL

Schools with educational and environmental interventions to increase water intake conducted a study involving German children. Researchers discovered that students had a lower risk of being overweight when they drank more water compared to students in schools that did not implement this intervention. Overall, students at the schools with the intervention drank 1.1 more glasses of water per day compared to the other school children.[7]

RAISE YOUR GLASS FOR A HAPPIER METABOLISM

Metabolism and water go together like—you guessed it—a wink and a smile. Your life is sustained with the energy from water and food. This process within the body is called *metabolism*. Increasing the body's metabolism can help you to lose weight and also prevent fat formation. Are you interested in how this happens? The liver carries on many functions, including fat metabolism. It will even take over part of the work when the kidneys are exhausted from not acquiring enough water to do their job. When this occurs, liver productivity diminishes, and there goes fat metabolism. Say good-bye to the happy moments on your bathroom scale.

The liver can focus on its basic functions and the kidneys can do their job when you fill up at the water cooler. Studies indicate that metabolism can increase by 30 percent when a person drinks at least eight glasses of water each day.[8] That is a major jump when looking to lose weight, so just think what can be accomplished when you drink the recommended eight glasses of water a day.

Water is key to flushing out toxins. Water transports sloughed-off fat cells, toxins, and waste products out of your body. It is also crucial for metabolizing fat in the liver. This translates to more efficient weight loss. The liver will just store the fat if it doesn't get plenty of water.

EIGHT WAYS WATER HELPS YOU LOSE WEIGHT

1. Energizes the body
2. Helps tone the muscles
3. Suppresses the appetite
4. Flushes toxins from the body
5. Improves digestion
6. Reduces cholesterol (start drinking more water instead of taking prescription drugs)
7. Stops the hunger-for-thirst confusion
8. Prevents bloating and water retention

PSST! WANT TO KNOW
WATER'S LITTLE SECRETS?

Science is just beginning to discover the fascinating story behind water. We tend to take water for granted because we know so little about it. We forget how vital it is to our health and often abuse and pollute it. Thousands of gallons of toxic chemicals are released into the ground and contaminate our water supply when we dig through the earth looking for natural resources, such as gas and oil. This process is called fracking. And pollution of our water certainly doesn't end there. From commercial factories to pesticides, chemicals seep into our groundwater daily.

Quantum physicists are beginning to unravel hidden mysteries about water. Oxygen and hydrogen atoms form energy bonds within water. This is one of its important secrets. The hydrogen-bond length of H_2O molecules is relatively weak. The electrostatic forces are affected in a way that alters the energy of electrons in your RNA. DNA information is transmitted into the cells by RNA, the carrier molecule, which in turn controls their chemical reactions.[9] This results in energy!

Energy is a coveted commodity when you are on a weight loss program. Energy fuel is produced in the little mitochondria of each of your cells. They produce ATP, your energy fuel. You will feel like a complete couch potato without energy fuel. When your cells are fired up, you feel like being productive, getting things done, taking the stairs instead of the elevator, exercising, or parking the car farther away from your destination. You have mental energy to figure out how to solve problems and order your day.

LOOK WHAT THEY'VE DONE
TO OUR WATER, MA!

A few years ago, Miley Cyrus recorded a remake of Melanie's 1971 hit, "Look What They've Done to My Song, Ma." We should all be singing, "Look what they've done to my water, Ma!" Throughout most of the United States, tap water (and bottled water that is sourced from tap) is laced with fluoride, chlorine, and an array of other chemicals. In some areas, water is contaminated with lead, such as in Flint, Michigan—a disaster only recently corrected. We just can't trust water from the tap these days.

There has been talk of fluoride being beneficial to your dental health, but this is just not the truth. It is a common misconception that fluoride prevents cavities. It is actually the exact opposite. Children in India were the basis of a 2011 study that illustrated how fluoride definitely does not fight cavities.[10] Fluoride is actually a toxin that can cause a wide range of health problems and leads to an increased risk of cavities. It accelerates aging due to cellular damage and weakens the immune system.[11]

Do you want to run the other way when you hear that something causes wrinkles? Look at fluoride; its use is associated with low thyroid function. It is a halogen that disrupts thyroid function and displaces iodine, a trace mineral so many people are already short on. This will result in weight gain. (Bromine and chlorine are also halogens.) Your ability to lose weight can be impeded by these toxins. The body protects organs by storing these bad guys in fat cells. Until you detox, the body will hold on to them. If you continue to bog down your body with these poisons, more fat cells will be created to store the toxic substances and protect your life. On top of all this, chlorine and other added chemicals cause tap water to taste awful.

CLEAN WATER: A KEY TO VIBRANT HEALTH

Hippocrates said fresh air and clean water were essential parts of good health.

We all know we should drink plenty of water. But toxins in many forms of water can make us sick. Scientific analysis of municipal drinking water has identified many new toxic contaminants. A landmark Associated Press investigation found that at least 41 million people drank water that contained trace amounts of pharmaceuticals, such as anticonvulsants, mood stabilizers, and sex hormones.

Among the non-prescription drugs detected were acetaminophen and ibuprofen: "Added to this are many known contaminants such as chlorine by-products, aluminum, industrial chemicals, pesticides, fluoride, lead, arsenic and naturally occurring radioactivity such as uranium."[12]

WHAT ABOUT GOVERNMENT STANDARDS?

Dr. Roy Speiser, a water quality specialist and health-care practitioner with more than three decades of experience in the field of environmental health, says people are being misled to believe that water is safe because it meets government standards. He comments: "If your local water report says the amount of a certain chemical is 'negligible' (whether it's true or not), consider what 'negligible' translates to over months and years of consumption."[13] In other words, chemicals and heavy metals keep accumulating until they reach toxic levels in the body and manifest as a health disorder.

FILTER YOUR WATER

Water purifiers to the rescue! Unless you have pure well water that has been proven free of contaminants, I recommend that you acquire a good water purifier, such as a distiller or a ceramic filter. However, a distiller will remove all the minerals in water. When detoxifying your body, distilled water is best; but otherwise, some minerals are beneficial to the body. Make sure you get a machine that removes most of the fluoride. Many water purifiers don't remove it because it is a difficult chemical to remove.

"Water filtration is essential," insists Dr. Speiser. He adds, "The more we continue to drink unfiltered water, the sicker we become, no matter what precautions we take in every other area of our life. Filtration is a measure both preventative and necessary. If you want to avoid illness, you cannot drink toxic water; if you are sick and want to get better, you cannot drink toxic water."[14] Conclusion: you cannot drink toxic water if you endeavor to be a healthy person free of disease.

"'A patient won't be able to undergo a thorough detoxification regimen if he or she is drinking unfiltered water,' explains Dr. Louis Vastola. 'While I am trying to restore healthy probiotics...the chlorine, fluoride, and ammonia in toxic water kill them off again, rendering the person's progress futile.' It only makes sense that true healing is dependent on the purity of the single most important carrying agent in our lives."[15]

DO YOUR MATH ON WATER

The body consists of 35–40 percent solid matter and 60–65 percent water. You must keep it well hydrated to maintain this ratio. We often wait until our mouths are dry to drink water, but by then we are already dehydrated. Don't wait until your mouth feels like a cotton ball to begin drinking water. Have some refreshing water long before that happens, and continue to drink it steadily throughout the day.

Some experts recommend taking your weight and dividing that number by two to determine the total number of ounces of water you should consume each day. Following that advice, you should drink about a gallon of water every day if you weigh two hundred pounds or more. If you usually don't drink a lot of water, this may sound like a daunting amount. Just begin with eight, eight-ounce glasses a day and steadily increase to the desired amount. You will be used to drinking the proper amount of water in about a week.

FLAVOR IT UP!

Drinking water all the time may seem boring to some people because it lacks flavor. A water purifier will enhance the taste, but if that just doesn't cut it, flavor it up. If lack of flavor is holding you back from getting your H_2O, get creative! Flavored water is not perfect, clear water, but at least you're drinking water. Infuse some natural flavorings, such as mint, lemon-ginger, cucumber, lemongrass, rosemary, or cranberry in your water. For example, try a splash of unsweetened cranberry juice in a big glass of water. A cup of hot water and lemon with a pinch of cayenne is a wonderful way to begin your day. This will jump-start your liver, which is very important for flushing toxins and metabolizing fat.

In chapter 8 I list a number of recipes for healthy and refreshing ways to tickle your taste buds. These fresh, fancy specialty waters are reminiscent of your favorite spa environment, and you can treat yourself to them right at home. In addition, cucumber, lemon, and cranberry are natural diuretics that will help you eliminate water weight and flush toxins and undesirable waste from your body. The body always eliminates water before body fat, so drink several glasses of cucumber, lemon, or cranberry water if it seems like you're retaining fluid. This will also assist you in eliminating toxins and help you feel more energized.

Keep in mind that you lose the cleansing properties required for health and weight loss when water is flavored, even naturally. Water takes on another message when something is added to it because it is an information carrier. The body now receives it as food. You need to drink several glasses of plain, pure water each day, even with your flavored water. So, chug-a-lug!

Give your body extra health benefits and kick up the flavor of your water with these creative water recipes:

ZESTY WATER

½ cucumber, sliced
1 handful fresh mint
1 lemon, sliced, peeled if not organic
1 Tbsp. grated fresh ginger

Put all ingredients in a pitcher and fill all the way up with pure water. Place it in the refrigerator for a few hours to make "Zesty Water," a scrumptious alternative to store-bought flavored waters.

HERE COMES THE SUN...WATER

Making sun water is the same concept as sun tea, minus the tea bags. Set a glass container filled with purified water out in the sun. By the end of the day, you will have vitamin D–infused sun water.[16]

ZERO-CALORIE AND FLAVORED WATERS

There are a variety of artificially sweetened waters with different flavors designed to take the place of soda. Research shows that artificial sweeteners actually cause people to gain more weight by causing people to eat more food. Zero calories in this case doesn't mean these waters are slimming.

GRAB YOUR WATER BOTTLE AND DRINK UP!

Water truly is life. The more we consume, the more alive we feel. We become refreshed, energized, and rinsed of residue. As our water intake increases, the body's craving for it increases. We begin to function in a greater sense of harmony. The benefits of water seem endless. Drinking it is one of the easiest ways we can lose weight and revitalize our entire being. So always have that water bottle close by and allow the amazing H_2O molecules to transform your body and mind.

CHAPTER 3

GAME CHANGERS: METABOLISM BOOSTERS AND WEIGHT LOSS HELPERS

A<small>RE YOU LOOKING</small> for some weight loss help beyond will-power, white knuckles, and good food choices? This chapter is for you. Boosting your metabolism may be a key for you. There is nothing splashy or fun to say about metabolism. It's the chemistry of the body—one reaction after another. But speeding it up can help you make a big splash in how you look at the next family reunion or holiday party.

Basically, the body's way of providing the energy it requires from food is referred to as *metabolism*. This biochemical process exists within all living organisms; it occurs to maintain life by permitting us to respond to our environment, repair damage, and grow. Sitting for an extended length of time and starvation dieting immensely decelerate your metabolism, while eating healthy foods, exercise, and adequate sleep are known to boost the metabolism.

WHAT DOES METABOLISM HAVE TO DO WITH WEIGHT?

Metabolism significantly influences your ability to lose weight. The amount of calories you burn during physical activity and at rest depends on your rate of metabolism, which is primarily determined by genetics. Some individuals have a slower or even lethargic metabolism and must be very aware of what they eat. Others have a naturally high metabolism and seem to be able to feast on high-calorie foods without gaining an ounce.

Though your genetic makeup is permanent, there are ways to change your metabolism and give it a boost in order to induce greater weight loss or sustain your current weight. Here are several pointers you can incorporate for success.

1. Increasing your muscle mass helps you lose weight. This means you will burn more calories even when you're not working out. Strength training is the key.

2. Keeping your blood sugar stable is very important. Make sure you are eating adequate protein and vegetables and not consuming sweets, which cause spikes and dips in blood sugar. If your blood sugar dips, then your brain sends a signal to eat more food. That's why stable blood sugar is so important.

3. Getting your ZZZs. You need seven (some say 7.5) to nine hours of rejuvenating sleep a night. There is a hormone called leptin that sends a message to the body when it has had enough to eat. Studies indicate that leptin levels lower when a person is sleep deprived. This interferes with the body's ability to regulate how much you eat. Cortisol is a stress hormone that interferes with your blood sugar control. When you suffer from sleep deprivation, your body will also produce more cortisol. It's the hormone that

is credited with depositing fat on the belly. There is also a hormone called ghrelin that promotes hunger; according to Harvard Health Publications, insufficient sleep can spike its levels.[1]

INCREASE YOUR BROWN FAT

The journal *Diabetes* published a notable study that proposes how a person's stores of brown fat, the "good fat," are stimulated by cooler temperatures, or simply by turning up the air conditioner. This burns through "bad" fat stores and assists in keeping us warm. Over a period of a few weeks, participants slept in bedrooms with various temperatures: a warm eighty-one degrees, a cool sixty-six degrees, and a mild-warm seventy-five degrees. Brown fat nearly doubled in the men who slept four weeks in sixty-six degrees. Now that's cool![2]

4. Getting plenty of H_2O. Water is the exciting miracle beverage when it comes to burning calories. Without enough water, you can't burn calories efficiently. Here is an easy way to keep track of how you're doing on the hydration front. Actually, no color—as in clear—urine is the best indicator of good hydration, although very light yellow is also good. (If you take B vitamins, it will color your urine bright yellow. If this is you, take a few days off from your supplement once in a while to see how well you are hydrating your body.)

    The Journal of Clinical Endocrinology and Metabolism published a study that depicted how the metabolic rates of its participants increased by 30 percent after drinking only two tall glasses (seventeen ounces) of water.[3]

5. Eating plenty of vegetables and fruits. The journal *PLOS Medicine* published a study where investigators surveyed weight changes and diet habits in more than 133,000 women and men for up to twenty-four years. Over a four-year time span the researchers discovered that eating more vegetables and fruit was linked to a higher rate of weight loss. Also, eating low-glycemic-index foods high in fiber—such as broccoli and brussels sprouts—in comparison to foods with a higher glycemic index was linked to increased weight loss.[4] Blending or juicing vegetables is one of the simplest methods to incorporate more of them in your diet. Even the veggies you don't like will mix right in with a delicious basic recipe. The taste will be masked by the scrumptious medley of vegetables and fruits that you do enjoy. Chances are, you won't even notice that they are there—but your body will be pleased with the nutrients.

6. Adding superfood metabolism boosters. That's a big part of this chapter, so read on. I also want to mention that I recommend a superfoods juice powder, Garden's Best Superfood Juice Powder, that you can just mix in water or juice. It really helps your metabolism.

PEOPLE LOSE FIVE TO TEN POUNDS AT OUR JUICE RETREATS

With every retreat we hold, people lose weight— usually five to ten pounds in a week. That's because we offer a three-day juice fast in the middle of the week that includes wheatgrass juice shots twice a day. We have plenty of metabolism boosters as part of the program. I want to share with you what one participant said.

JAY LOST TEN POUNDS

"The Juice Retreat has definitely changed my life. I have lost over ten pounds. The amount of knowledge that you have shared with us will take us a long way."

THE VEGETABLES, FRUIT, SPICES, HERBS, AND TEAS THAT HELP YOU LOSE WEIGHT

When you incorporate these foods into your juices and blended drinks, you will help to boost your metabolism and promote weight loss. The drink, soup, and smoothie recipes on the following pages are all listed in chapter 8.

VEGETABLES

Asparagus

The *West Indian Medical Journal* published a study in 2010 that showed how asparagus can operate as a natural diuretic.[5] This is especially beneficial for people who suffer from high blood pressure and edema because it helps the body dispose of excess fluid and salt. It also assists in preventing kidney stones, as it flushes out toxins from the kidneys. Try the Asparagus Limeade recipe.

Celery

Celery is known as a thermogenic food. Significant levels of calcium are found in this common vegetable. Celery also has diuretic properties that stimulate the flow of urine from the body. This causes metabolism to increase and bloating to decrease, as well as breaking down fat cells more efficiently.[6] Refer to the recipe Celery Delight.

Cucumber

High amounts of sulfur and silicon are found in cucumbers, which promotes the elimination of uric acids. This provides relief from bloating and feeling overstuffed. It also creates an efficient system of waste removal from the body. Make the Cucumber Siesta.

Red cabbage

Cabbage accelerates your body's production of two hormones—leptin (appetite suppressing) and adiponectin (fat burning). This results in a higher degree of weight loss. An array of essential minerals is also found in red cabbage: copper, calcium, selenium, potassium, magnesium, iron, phosphorous, manganese, and zinc. Try the Red Cabbage Cocktail.

Watercress

A study from the United Kingdom proves watercress's effectiveness in weight loss. The focus of the diet involved a soup made with watercress. Eleven volunteers who followed this diet for six weeks lost an average of one stone (fourteen pounds); one man lost 3.5 stone (forty-nine pounds), including nearly 10 percent of his body fat.

The diet's simplicity impressed all the participants. Within the first week almost everyone lost weight, which amped up the motivation of the group. Weight loss was only one of the benefits. Everyone remarked how their hair and skin had improved and that "they felt unusually energized."[7]

As mentioned in the introduction, I conducted a similar study with fifty-five female volunteers in which 51 percent lost between four and six pounds in the first week on the Watercress Soup and

Smoothie Diet. By three weeks nearly half the participants had lost between six and nine pounds. The good thing about watercress is that it provides nutrients without a significant addition of calories. Considered the top superfood, this aquatic plant is one of the most nutrient-dense vegetables known to man. I believe this is one of the reasons many of the women that participated in my Watercress Soup Diet said they were not hungry after eating a bowl of this soup. In fact, many of them said cravings just disappeared. See the Watercress Weight Loss Soup recipe.

Melissa Lost Six Pounds

I am down six pounds, my skin is softer, and I have lots of energy too. I believe that the iodine from [the watercress] is doing wonders for me. I usually just take [an iodine] supplement in pill form. My numbers have always been in the "normal" range when my thyroid is tested; however, I seem to experience some of the symptoms of a thyroid issue. I was also tested for diabetes and my A1c was elevated and in the prediabetic range. It has stayed the same for the past two times I went in. I am curious to see if this diet will change that!! I am very optimistic! Oh, one more thing I noticed is that the redness where my incisions were for shoulder surgery I had done at the end of March is going away! The color has faded to a very light pink, and the tenderness at the incisions is gone too.

Watercress benefits workouts

While working out, watercress has also proven very beneficial. Exercise is at the base of developing a strong metabolism. In one research study, ten healthy young men received about three ounces of watercress. For eight weeks, these participants engaged in workouts on a treadmill. Their routine included intense exercise in short bursts. As a control, another group implemented the eight-week workout without the use of watercress. Those who ingested watercress revealed benefits after a single dose. The athletes who did not consume watercress experienced more DNA damage. The nutrients responded on the spot and did not require any length of time to build up in the system. The participants who ate the veggie daily for two months reaped identical benefits as those who ingested it only two hours before getting on the treadmill the first time.[8]

Thyroid rescue

Thyroid function is also improved by watercress. Studies indicate that consistent consumption of watercress has benefits that may be from "secondary metabolites and other phytonutrients, which repair cellular damage." They operate efficiently as a preventive agent against cardiovascular disease, thyroid disease, and some cancers. Watercress is also one of the vegetables with the highest amounts of iodine, which is very important for your thyroid.[9]

Watercress face-lift

On top of all of this, you can appear younger while you drop the weight! A study conducted with the watercress diet proves this to be true. An article in the *Daily Mail*—the UK's second-best-selling newspaper—called watercress "the latest wonder food" for the face and raved about its antiaging abilities. Ten out of eleven women who went on the watercress diet experienced visible regeneration in their skin, and seven of eleven saw improvement in their wrinkles. The story also mentioned that watercress contains more vitamin C than oranges and four times more beta-carotene and vitamin A than apples, tomatoes, and broccoli.[10] Taste the Energizing Watercress Cocktail.

Wheatgrass juice

Selenium is crucial for the healthy functioning of the thyroid gland, and it is prevalent in wheatgrass. Impaired thyroid function, even when it is linked to autoimmune diseases and other issues, can be improved by adding selenium to your diet, according to a 2017 study published in *International Journal of Endocrinology*.[11] Weight loss efforts progress as your thyroid function improves. An article on wheatgrass juice was published in 2002 by the *International Journal of Obesity and Related Metabolic Disorders*. It mentioned that researchers discovered that wheatgrass is beneficial for fighting type 2 diabetes and obesity. It contains phytanic acid, which is a chlorophyll-derived metabolite that attacks fat cells and type 2 diabetes and is useful in the treatment of obesity.[12]

FRUIT

Avocado

Avocados have a lovable, buttery consistency. When it comes to thickening a smoothie, they are more ideal than sugar-rich bananas. *Nutrition Journal* released a survey that indicated how consuming a medium-sized avocado per day can decrease one's odds of developing metabolic syndrome by 50 percent and improve overall diet quality. Avocado aficionados also report a slimmer waist circumference and lower body mass index (BMI).[13] The survey also reported that participants who ate half a fresh avocado at lunch reported a 40 percent reduction in appetite.[14] Blended drinks and smoothies are awesome with an avocado. Try the Rockin' Green Smoothie recipe.

Blueberry and mulberry

Berries are rich in anthocyanin. They have been proven to lower cholesterol levels among rats fed with a HFD (high-fat diet), reduce insulin resistance, and inhibit weight gain.[15] Enjoy the Mulberry Hemp Smoothie.

Cranberry juice

Urinary tract infections are traditionally treated with cranberry juice. This is because of its diuretic and antibacterial properties. Drink Cranberry Apple Delight.

Grapefruit

The journal *Metabolism* says that eating a grapefruit prior to a meal for only six weeks diminished waist size by up to an inch. Scientists credit grapefruit's powerful fat-melting effects to its phytochemicals.

If you are on any medications, check with your doctor first, because grapefruit can have some adverse effects when mixed with prescriptions. If your physician says it is safe to proceed, then you can begin to reap the benefits by enjoying half of a grapefruit before breakfast. Or you can juice it up. You can also add a few segments of this fruit to your salads.[16]

One study of ninety-one obese patients separated them into four different groups. Each group was given one of the following: 1) half a fresh grapefruit with a placebo capsule, 2) grapefruit juice and placebo capsules, 3) grapefruit capsules and apple juice, or 4) placebo capsules and apple juice. In just twelve weeks, every group that had grapefruit in their systems saw significant weight loss compared to the group that took just the placebos. The most important improvement in insulin resistance occurred with the patients in the group that consumed the half fresh grapefruit. They also experienced the highest increase in weight loss.[17] Try the Grapefruit Fennel Jicama Cocktail listed in chapter 8.

Lemon

Lemon contains d-limonene, which helps reduce bloating. Since ancient times this phytonutrient found in citrus rind oil has been utilized for its diuretic effects. Scientific findings supporting these claims were recently discovered. The *Journal of the Pharmaceutical Society of Japan* published an animal study that proved bloat due to water retention can be diminished by d-limonene.[18] Taste the Lemon Berry Limeade.

Tomato

In an eight-week study, thirty female participants with a BMI greater than 20 supplemented their normal diets with 280 milliliters (mL) of tomato juice. The findings concluded that supplementing tomato juice greatly decreased cholesterol levels, body weight, waist circumference, BMI, and body fat.[19] Enjoy the Lively Tomato Lemon Smoothie.

SPICES

Black pepper

Fat-burning properties are characteristic of black pepper (as well as ginger). The formation of new fat cells has also been shown to be blocked by use of this spice. This impedes weight gain from the very beginning. You can sprinkle black pepper on virtually everything; it is even tasty on foods that are traditionally sweeter, such as oatmeal, yogurt, or smoothies. Try the Spice It Up Smoothie recipe.

Cinnamon

Cinnamon imitates the action of insulin in the body, therefore regulating the effects of sugar levels. Glucose's metabolism is improved twentyfold due to this "insulin-like" activity.[20] Excess sugar in your blood is converted into fatty acids by the liver. The metabolism of blood sugar increases and energy is created when cinnamon is ingested. Taste Cinnamon Swirl, a tasty treat made with coconut milk.

Chili peppers

A compound found in chili peppers, capsaicin, is responsible for enhancing metabolism. A study on its effects discovered that it has a high inhibitory effect against fat storage. Capsaicin enhances the breakdown of fats and suppresses inflammatory responses, preventing obesity-induced insulin resistance.[21] Try the Spicy Cacao Smoothie.

Cumin

A recent study performed on overweight women revealed that you can burn up to three times more body fat by adding one teaspoon of cumin to a recipe.[22] Try Energizing Carrot Cumin Cold Soup.

Ginger

A study published in *Metabolism* determined that drinking two grams of ginger powder in hot water reduced hunger cravings. Participants who didn't drink the ginger water were hungrier after a three-hour time span.[23] To see its effects, try the Ginger Helper recipe.

Turmeric

Curcumin is the active compound found in turmeric. The journal *BioFactors* illustrated how curcumin transforms the composition of fatty cells into calorie-burning cells.[24] This offers a good option for overweight and obese individuals. Taste the Turmeric Twister.

COOL LITTLE FOOD TIP!

Mix mustard into your meal and kill off the calories. Eating one teaspoon of mustard (about five calories) can boost metabolism by up to 25 percent for several hours—a discovery made by scientists at England's Oxford Polytechnic Institute. Researchers credit the benefits to the phytochemicals allyl isothiocyanate and capsaicin, which give mustard its distinctive taste.[25]

HERBS

Dandelions

The dandelion plant is growing in popularity due to its array of health benefits. Its days of being considered only a pesky weed by gardeners is over. This so-called weed increases your intake of vitamins E, C, and A, as well as minerals such as potassium and iron. It also helps to reduce bloating and increases weight loss.[26] Research also concludes that dandelion has a diuretic effect by increasing urination.[27] Try the Dandelion Lime Elixir.

Garlic

Despite causing stinky breath, juicing or eating more of this herb may assist your body in burning fat. One study discovered that mice that ate garlic lost more weight in seven weeks than mice that did not have garlic in their diets.[28] Try making Garlic Love. (Eating some parsley after ingesting garlic will help take away "garlic breath.")

Parsley

One study showed substantial evidence for the diuretic effect of parsley. According to the study, "Rats offered an aqueous parsley seed extract to drink, eliminated a significantly larger volume of urine per 24 [hours] as compared to when they were drinking water."[29] Try Parsley Pep.

TEAS

Ashwagandha tea

Ashwagandha diminishes stress hormones that expand your waistline, and creates a brighter outlook on life. The *Indian Journal of Psychological Medicine* released a study that indicates that ashwagandha root extract effectively improves an individual's resistance toward stress and improves one's perception of life. Stress is certainly not an ally, especially when one is aiming to lose weight.[30] In a recent Penn State University study, increased levels of inflammation were found in the bodies of people who reacted poorly to high-stress situations. Inflammation is also directly linked to cancer, diabetes, heart disease, and obesity. Stress hormones such as cortisol (the belly fat hormone) are heightened in high-anxiety situations. Cortisol draws lipids from the bloodstream and stores them in fat cells.[31]

Barberry tea

Berberine is a naturally occurring, powerful, fat-fighting chemical found in the root bark, fruit, and stem of the barberry shrub. Chinese researchers conducted a study of how berberine prevents the development of insulin resistance in rats that consume a high-fat diet. It can also prevent weight gain. Prior studies also indicate that ingesting barberry can diminish the amount of receptors on the surface of fat cells and boost energy expenditure. This makes fat-promoting foods from incoming sources less likely to be absorbed.[32]

Goji tea

Goji berries are harvested from a plant called *Lycium barbarum*. Diabetes and other diseases are traditionally treated with this Asian medicinal therapy. It has slimming effects. Participants in a study published by the *Journal of the American College of Nutrition* were given either a placebo or a single dose of L. barbarum after finishing a meal. One hour after taking the dose, researchers noted that the placebo group was burning calories at a rate 10 percent lower than the goji berry group; these results continued for up to four hours. For an extra bonus, green tea is mixed in with most goji teas, causing calories to burn at an even higher rate.[33]

Green tea

Fat literally melts away with the use of green tea because it is replete with catechins, which contain fat-burning properties. Epigallocatechin gallate (EGCG) is a specific group of the antioxidant compounds found in green tea. These compounds increase the release of fat from cells (specifically in the belly), accelerate the metabolism, and help in reducing adipose tissue. The liver's fat burning capacity also speeds up. There is even more great news. Exercise combined with the regular consumption of green tea maximizes weight loss benefits. Researchers conducted a study where participants engaged in a twenty-minute workout. The ones who drank four to five cups of green tea a day lost two more pounds than the people who did not drink green tea.[34]

Hawthorn berry

This berry is related to the rose family and is a mighty diuretic. It lessens symptoms of congestive heart failure, as it reduces any buildup of fluid. Urinary flow and excretion is also heightened by this plant's nutritious value. Kidney problems may also be alleviated by the hawthorn berry.[35]

Hibiscus

According to a 2012 study, there are valid diuretic effects in the roselle species of hibiscus.[36] Greater filtration through the kidneys was also documented in another study involving hibiscus.[37]

Horsetail

According to a study conducted in 2014, prescription diuretics function in the same fashion as horsetail extract, but the diuretics come with side effects. If you have been plagued with side effects from pharmaceutical diuretics, horsetail may provide a solution.[38]

Juniper

The juniper plant has been used as a diuretic since medieval times. Its benefits have seldom been recorded in modern-day studies, but the volume of urine in animals has been significantly affected by this evergreen. Potassium levels are not lowered by this natural diuretic as they are with some prescription drugs.

Matcha

Matcha means "powdered tea." It has amazing health benefits. It is a derivative of the Japanese tencha leaf and is stone ground into a fine powder. The EGCG concentrate found in matcha out-numbers the typical green tea by 137 times. A dieter and EGCG are the best of buddies. Research has indicated that matcha can con-currently obstruct the formation of fat cells (adipogenesis) and raise the breakdown of fat (lipolysis), especially in the stomach region. A study documented that men who consumed green tea with 136 mg EGCG, which is the equivalent of an individual four-gram serving of matcha, lost double the weight of the placebo group (5.3 pounds versus 2.8 pounds lost) and quadruple the amount of belly bulge over a three-month time span. The powder may be traditionally prepared in the ancient style of the Zen monks, which dates back to AD 1191, or savored in smoothies, iced drinks, milkshakes, or lattes, which is in conjunction with the new wave of superfoods. As an additional benefit, four grams of protein—more than the amount found in an egg white—are hidden within a single serving of matcha.[39]

Oolong tea

Drinking oolong tea can also give your metabolism a jolt. The body's ability to metabolize fat increases, which increases weight loss. The metabolism-boosting effects are attributed to the catechins found in oolong. This is the same case with green tea. Participants in a study published by the *Chinese Journal of Integrative Medicine* reported that over a six-week time span, those who regularly sipped oolong tea lost six pounds.[40]

Pu-erh tea

Fat cells virtually shrivel when you drink this fermented Chinese tea. Chinese researchers separated rats into five groups and over a two-month period fed them various diets. Three groups ate varying doses of pu-erh tea extract along with a high-fat diet, one group ate a high-fat diet with no tea supplementation, and one group was served as the control group. The research concluded that the pu-erh tea drastically lowered potentially hazardous fat located in the blood, known as triglyceride concentrations. The groups with the high-fat diet that had the tea also showed a reduction in belly fat. The outcome in humans may vary slightly, though these findings are significant enough to acknowledge. Prepare yourself a piping hot cup and experience the benefits.[41]

Rooibos tea

The "red bush" plant produces leaves that make rooibos tea. It is grown solely near Cape Town in the Cederberg region of South Africa. The powerful and unique flavonoid aspalathin makes rooibos tea particularly great for your flattening your belly. South African researchers stated that flavonoids and polyphenols inhibit the formation of new fat cells by as much as 22 percent. This process is called adipogenesis. Fat metabolism is also supported by these chemicals.[42]

White tea

Nutrition and Metabolism released a study that showed how white tea amplifies the body's ability to utilize and break down existing fat for energy. It even prevents new fat cells from forming. In addition, says the study's author, Elma Baron, MD, "Chemicals in the tea appear to protect your skin from sun-induced stress, which can cause the cells to break down and age prematurely."[43] Before applying sunblock, use a lotion infused with white tea to experience the benefits.

Yerba maté

Yerba maté's impressive thermogenic effects accelerate your body's calorie-burning mechanism. It improves insulin sensitivity, therefore inducing weight loss. One study assembled two groups of participants. Sixty minutes prior to exercising, group one took a 1,000 milligram (mg) capsule of yerba maté and group two ingested a placebo. The study concluded that the beneficial effects the workout had on the participants' metabolisms were increased by the consumption of this herb.[44] In addition, it supplies plenty of chromium, which helps stabilize blood sugar levels. It has a cache of B-vitamins and 90 percent more powerful cancer fighting antioxidants than other teas.

MORE HELP FOR THAT CREEPING SCALE

Apple cider vinegar

Apple cider vinegar has a long history of helping people find better health. Hippocrates commonly prescribed it for an array of ailments. Suggested for alleviating the symptoms of diabetes, arthritis, and muscle aches and pains, recent studies have proven it will even facilitate weight loss. The *Journal of Agriculture and Food Chemistry* published a study where mice were fed acetic acid (the key component of vinegar) along with a high-fat diet. Their body fat decreased 10 percent more than the rodents in the control group. This led researchers to believe that genes that trigger enzymes are propelled by acetic acid. This prevents weight gain and breaks down fat.[45]

In 2009, scientists from Japan undertook an investigation to determine this effect on humans, conducting a double-blind trial on obese adults with similar waist measurements and body weights. Researchers assembled three groups of participants. A beverage consisting of half an ounce of apple cider vinegar (ACV) was consumed by one of the groups for twelve weeks; another group consumed one ounce of apple cider vinegar. A third group consumed a drink that did not contain apple cider vinegar. People consuming the beverages containing ACV experienced decreased BMI and body weight, and reduced waist measurements and triglycerides, in comparison to those who did not drink the apple cider vinegar.[46]

Coconut water

Pure coconut water is a wonderful choice for replacing electrolytes, especially if you have been working out or sweating profusely. It is the highest known source of electrolytes. Around the world there are remote areas that administer coconut juice intravenously for short intervals. This assists in emergency situations that involve dehydrated patients. However, it is wise to refrain from drinking more than one eight-ounce serving a day because of its high carb content.

BEVERAGES TO AVOID

Soft drinks

The negative repercussions of drinking soda pop seem to go on forever, with its highly fattening qualities only the beginning. If you suffer from any degree of stiffness, arthritis, weight problems, fibromyalgia, rheumatism—or, frankly, you just value your health— you cannot risk consuming any form of soda. It is jam-packed with toxic chemicals, overloaded with sugar or artificial sweeteners, and highly acidic. Avoid them like the plague. If you experience pains and muscle aches, or suffer from cancer or fibromyalgia, such avoidance is even more crucial. An acidic body (which can be caused by soda) will magnify these ailments. Drinking soft drinks makes weight loss extremely difficult; weight gain will most likely be the outcome. Soda also has addictive ingredients. It is brimming with phosphorous, which robs the bones of calcium. You may develop osteoporosis, thus crippling you for life.

The soda industry has produced massive amounts of advertising and propaganda that suggest substituting diet drinks for sugary drinks will inhibit weight gain. This is simply not true. It has been proven that diet soda is even more fattening than regular sodas. Diet drinks have also been found to be worse for your health than sugar-sweetened soda. A study of more than 66,000 women conducted over a fourteen-year period supports this conclusion. These facts may influence us all to boycott diet products for life. The study found:

- Sugar-sweetened sodas cause less risk of diabetes than diet sodas.

- Risk of type 2 diabetes increased by 33 percent in women who consumed one twelve-ounce soda per week, and the risk increased by 66 percent in women who consumed one twenty-ounce soda per week.

- Artificial sweeteners are more addictive than sugar, and women who drank artificially sweetened sodas consumed twice as many. Regular sugar is also hundreds to thousands of times less sweet. Regardless of a person's body weight, artificial sweeteners increased the risk of diabetes.[47]

Replacing soda pop with water, cranberry water, or lemon water is the best option. Purchase carbonated mineral water if you enjoy the bubbles. Jazz it up with a splash of fruit juice such as cranberry, green apple, lime, or lemon. Make delicious ginger ale by adding fresh ginger to apple juice and sparkling water. Your body will thank you for making a healthy choice. Some minor "withdrawal symptoms" may occur when you first eliminate soft drinks, but they will soon diminish without causing any harm. If symptoms occur, it's a sign that the body is relinquishing its addiction to artificial sweeteners and sugar. It is purging the toxins that were destroying it.

Vitamin water—almost as unhealthy as soda

One of the soda industry's biggest scams is vitamin water. It takes advantage of the public's inclining interest in healthy alternatives to soda. These drinks come nowhere near the mineral and vitamin content found in food. Vitamin water is actually one of the unhealthiest water choices available![48] Health-harming additives, such as the high-fructose corn syrup I mentioned in chapter 1, are found in most vitamin waters. This ingredient is the primary cause of diabetes, obesity, and metabolic syndrome. These waters also contain food dyes that destroy your emotional and physical health. Always select pure water in place of vitamin water.

Electrolyte and sports drinks

Brominated vegetable oil is an ingredient in most of these popular drinks. Bromine is a halogen that deteriorates thyroid health and interferes with the absorption of iodine. Acidity is also very high in these drinks. Soft drinks have two-thirds less sugar than most sports drinks. HFCS, which scars the liver, is also typically found in these drinks. If that weren't bad enough, there are also food colorings and artificial flavors in them, which produce ill health. They also contain excessive amounts of processed salt (sodium). Artificial sweeteners may be found in the products that are labeled "sugar free." This is even worse than HFCS.

Meal replacement drinks

Commercially sold meal replacement drinks consist of mostly sugar and water. The top four ingredients are maltodextrin (sugar), corn syrup, sugar, and water. They are also fortified with synthetic minerals and vitamins.

Alcohol

There are numerous reasons to avoid hard liquor, beer, and wine. Here is a new one you may not have heard before: When the body ingests alcohol, the pituitary gland will suppress secretion of the hormone vasopressin. A lack of this hormone leads to general dehydration. Your brain cells are even affected; inflammation and severe dehydration are caused by habitual use of caffeine and alcohol. If you occasionally indulge in this beverage, it is a good rule of thumb to chase every alcoholic drink with two glasses of water. Energy fuel–producing units (mitochondria) are also damaged by alcohol. With all of this information, you are now well aware of the significance of energy fuel and hydration. So, pass on that beer or wine you may be accustomed to enjoying and stick with a strategic weight loss program. Trust me. It pays off.

THE FINAL SIP

You can enjoy a wide range of beverages that will help you lose weight and improve your health. Try to include a wide variety of the ingredients highlighted in this chapter for maximum benefits with your Sipping Skinny Program.

CHAPTER 4

JUICING IT UP!

T HOUGH THIS ISN'T just a book about fresh juice, juice is still a big part of everything I do. After all, I am known as The Juice Lady. I continually hear from people who are new to juicing who have lots of questions: Is there protein in juice? Am I losing most of my nutrients when the fiber is ejected? If I wash my produce well, will I get rid of the pesticides? If you are new to juicing or you'd just like to know a little more about the subject, this chapter is for you.

Fresh juice is your delicious go-to drink for optimal health and efficient weight loss—a garden in your glass! Pour yourself a tall one and enjoy a natural vitamin-mineral potion with a bounty of nutrients and then revel in the happy results. "What results?" you might ask. Juice promotes weight loss and greater energy and vitality. But that's not all. Benefits from juice abound—it's health on a mission to rejuvenate your body. You may be surprised to discover all the different nutrients in juice, including protein, carbohydrates, essential fatty acids, enzymes, and phytonutrients. Researchers are continually studying juices' components to understand in more detail how these miracle substances help the body heal, maintain health, and help you shed those unwanted pounds.

So let's get started and discuss the wonderful benefits juice provides.

work together to make reactions happen. It is the flavonoids that make vitamin C more effective.

Minerals

Just like its abundance of vitamins, fresh juice is loaded with minerals. To function properly, our bodies rely on about two dozen minerals for healthy metabolism. Calcium, chloride, magnesium, phosphorus, potassium, sodium, and sulfur are among the major minerals. We also need trace minerals; as the name implies, we only need small amounts of them. Some of the trace minerals we need are boron, chromium, cobalt, copper, fluoride, manganese, nickel, selenium, vanadium, and zinc. Minerals and vitamins are components of enzymes. They are also part of bone, teeth, and blood tissues. They are critical in the maintenance of normal cellular function.

Minerals are found in inorganic forms in the soil. It is not until plants pull them from the earth through their small roots and incorporate them into their tissues that they become organic and usable by the human body. The minerals combine with organic molecules, which then transform them into absorbable forms of minerals. This is one of the important reasons we should eat our vegetables. Did you know that juice is believed to provide better mineral absorption than eating whole vegetables? Why? Juicing releases minerals into a highly absorbable state that is easily digested.

Enzymes

Enzymes are known as "living" molecules. Fresh juice is brimming with them. Their special job is to work with vitamins and minerals to speed up necessary reactions in our bodies that are vital for optimal health. In fact, enzymes are so necessary, we would not have life in our cells without them.

How we prepare our juice makes a difference. Enzymes are abundant in raw food, but they are destroyed easily by heat in cooking and the process of pasteurization. Bottled juices you buy in the market (even those found in the refrigerated section) are required to be pasteurized. Unfortunately, the required temperatures for pasteurization are far above the limit of what would preserve the enzymes, biophotons, and vitamins.

When you juice or eat raw food, these enzyme-rich foods are used to help break down proteins, carbs, and fats in the digestive tract. This spares the body's enzyme producers—the pancreas, stomach, and small intestines—from having to overwork. This is called the "law of adaptive secretion of digestive enzymes." Basically, this means the enzymes in your food help your body to secrete less of its own enzymes for digestion, whereby it is freed to focus on other functions such as repair, removal of dead and damaged cells, and rejuvenation. Therefore, fresh juices help the body function better by requiring less energy expenditure for digestion. When people drink fresh juice on a regular basis, they often report they experience more energy right away. I also frequently hear them report better brain function and the disappearance of pain.

Phytochemicals

This word is constructed of two words—*phyto*, meaning "plant," and *chemical*, which in this context means "nutrient." Basically, this means the plants contain substances that protect them from disease, injury, and pollution. It is from the phytochemicals (a.k.a. phytonutrients) that a plant receives color, odor, and flavor. Pick a variety of plant foods we typically eat and you will be amazed to learn there are tens of thousands of different types of phytochemicals in them! For example, the tomato. It may contain up to ten thousand individual phytochemicals, including lycopene, the best-known of its natural chemicals. Unlike vitamins and enzymes, phytochemicals are not destroyed by cooking.

Drinking vegetable juice is a great way to incorporate a large number of concentrated phytochemicals into your diet, and there is a very good reason to do this. According to research, people who regularly ingest a variety of phytochemicals have the lowest incidence of cancer and other diseases.

Biophotons

Basically, this word means "the light emitted biologically." Within the cells of raw fruits and vegetables we find a store of light energy. This energy is more difficult to measure than other nutrients. However, it is interesting to note that biophotons emit coherent light energy when a special photography process called Kirlian photography is used to reveal it. When we consume plant food, we are receiving this amazing light energy into our cells. Now scientists are discovering its many health benefits. Some of the benefits that researchers believe we receive through biophotons include aid to cellular communication, increase in our energy, physical and mental strength, and a feeling of well-being.

The word *vitalism* was used to discuss this essence before scientists researched biophotons. It means a vital spark or energy. The study of vitalism as a hypothesis dates back from the seventeenth to nineteenth centuries. There is also a long history of vitalism in medical philosophies, and it has been included for quite some time in the traditional healing practices. The professionals in this camp who studied disease believed its root cause was some imbalance of the vital energies (vital force) in the body.

Medical practices began to change and become more mechanistic in the twentieth century. This meant the focus on vitalism, or the vital spark of life, was basically discarded. But we cannot discard the vital spark, or biophotons. Through raw fruits and vegetables our bodies receive this vital life. This is one reason why so many people notice an increase of energy directly related to when they started juicing fruits and vegetables. You can usually spot people who juice; they look more radiant and have a healthy glow about them.

THE MOST COMMONLY ASKED QUESTIONS ABOUT JUICING

Do you have a few questions about the whole juicing process, like storage, fiber, or just how expensive it is? Read on. I've collected questions from many people through the years. I'll bet some of them are yours. My list continues to grow, but what follows are the questions I've been asked most often.

Is it expensive to juice?

It isn't cheap, but it usually costs less than buying your favorite fancy coffee drink. For example, if you make a juice of two carrots, half of a lemon, a bit of gingerroot, two ribs of celery, and a half of a cucumber, you will probably spend between $2 and $3.50. This will depend on sales, the store or farmer's market you choose, the area of the country where you live, and the time of year. It is cheaper if the produce is local and in season rather than shipped across the country and/or out of season.

To balance the cost scale, factor in the positive changes that will accompany your new juicing lifestyle. You most likely will no longer need as many vitamin supplements. You may not even need such over-the-counter medications as painkillers, sleeping aids, antacids, laxatives, and cold, cough, and flu medications. As your health improves and you experience less sickness, you'll be saving money. And depending on how much you save on this end, your juice may not cost you much at all. You may experience less lost time from work. Then you won't need to worry about running out of sick days and not getting paid for your time off. If you're self-employed, you won't miss out on income lost due to illness. Juicing helps you stay well all year long. What is that worth? Wouldn't you agree that bolstering your body with immune-building, disease-fighting vitamins and minerals from juicing translates into financial benefits, along with a host of other great benefits?

Juicing removes fiber. Is this an issue?

No. Yes, we need the insoluble fiber, but since we are combining eating high-fiber foods with juicing, we can still get our insoluble fiber from whole vegetables, fruits, sprouts, legumes, and whole grains. So no, it isn't an issue when you eat high-fiber foods. Juicing is then a supplement to your high-fiber diet.

It is important to remember that whole fruits and vegetables contain both soluble and insoluble fiber; we need both types for colon health. When juicing, the insoluble fiber is removed. However, soluble fiber remains in the forms of gums and pectin. Soluble fiber is quite beneficial for the digestive tract. It lowers blood cholesterol, stabilizes blood sugar, and improves good bacteria in the bowel. So don't worry about losing fiber. Instead, think about all the extra nutrients you are getting in this concentration of juice.

Some people are keeping the fiber in the juice. The new term I use is "souping." Blenders such as the Ninja and Vitamix have made blending vegetables and fruit very popular, hence the latest name and craze for blended drinks. So this is an option as well. (For more information, see my book *Souping Is the New Juicing*.)

I've heard that lots of nutrients are lost with the fiber. Is this true?

There was a time when people believed this, but this theory no longer holds water. The US Department of Agriculture did a study analyzing twelve fruits that had been juiced. They discovered that more than 90 percent of the nutrients remained in the juice, not with the fiber, once again proving that juice is a great supplement for the diet.[1]

Your main goal with juicing is to receive extra nutrients directly from food and not just from a vitamin pill, because food is better than a pill. In fact, juicing is one of the best sources of nutrients to bolster your vitamin and mineral intake. The additional vitamins and minerals will reduce your need for as many supplements, improve your health, and save you money. For help with juice as therapy, I recommend you read my book *The Juice Lady's Guide to Juicing for Health*.

I'm confused. Why not just eat fruits and vegetables instead of juicing them?

This isn't an either/or issue. I won't tell you to stop eating fruits and vegetables and just juice. However, let me give you three reasons why juicing is an important part of a healthy diet.

1. When we drink fresh juice, we are receiving the health benefits of many more fruits and vegetables than we could eat in a day. Chewing is good for you; however, trying to chew the equivalent of all the produce that goes into a juice recipe takes a lot longer than you might think.

   Are you just a bit curious about the time factor? I ran a simple experiment. I timed how long it would take me to eat the five medium-sized carrots that I can juice in less than a minute. Of course, my juice recipe also contained cucumber, lemon, gingerroot, beet, kale, and celery, but I only timed the carrots. It took me about fifty minutes to properly chew and consume those carrots. I don't have that kind of free time every day. And I had to laugh. When I was finished, my jaw was so tired and sore that I could hardly open my mouth. I didn't want to do that again.

2. Most of us don't eat the stems, leaves, and seeds of most produce, but when we juice, we can take advantage of those often-discarded parts. I do this. I juice beet stems and leaves; celery leaves; the pith (the white inside of the peel) of lemons, limes, and oranges; the seeds of lemons, apples, cucumbers, and watermelon; tough sections of asparagus and broccoli stems; and kale leaves with the ribs. Juicing allows us to waste not!

3. There is less digestive work for the body, since juicing has already broken down the food. Thus, juice starts nourishing the body quicker; in about twenty to thirty minutes it is believed to be at work in the body. The benefits are even more evident when the body is struggling with an ailment. Juicing relieves a lot of the work normally required for the digestive process.

juicer is inefficient and leaves wet pulp behind, or if the rpm is too high, you will end up wasting a lot of produce.

There are so many different juicers on the market. How do I know which one is best?

I've received hundreds of emails asking which juicer is best—cold press, masticating, or centrifugal. I consider a juicer a "must have" for a healthy kitchen, precisely because it separates juice from the fiber. Then there's nothing to slow down that veggie juice from getting into your system; it goes right to work, rejuvenating and healing your body. A juicer separates the fiber from the juice, which is what you want in this case.

There are two categories of juicers: cold press (masticating) and centrifuge.

Cold press (a.k.a. masticating) juicers

The cold press or masticating juicers press or crush produce to extract the juice. I know of one study showing that this type of juicer preserves a few more nutrients than the centrifuge juicers. Most masticating juicers will make wheatgrass juice, and they juice greens better than a centrifuge juice. They don't produce as much heat when processing and don't oxidize the juice as much; therefore, they preserve the vitamins and enzymes better.

The primary drawback of these "slow juicers" (as they are also called) revolves around time. Few of them have wide mouths, but even with the slow press juicers that do, you have to cut everything in small pieces—unlike the centrifuge juicers, which take most items whole. They are also slower than the centrifuge type. If time is your main issue and you don't have a lot of that precious commodity, then go for the centrifuge.

Centrifuge juicers

Most centrifuge juicers have wide mouths. They spin and separate juice from fiber by bursting cells open. They are faster to use because you don't have to cut most of your produce up, and they are speedier at the juicing process. I have that type and am very happy because I can juice and wash the juicer in about five minutes rather than spending about twenty minutes preparing juice. The drawback is the fast-spinning blade, which can generate heat and also oxidize the juice, thus destroying some of the vitamins and enzymes.

How do I choose the right juicer for me?

If fast is most important, even though you may lose a few more nutrients, this will still be the healthiest thing on earth you could drink. If time is of the essence to you, then you might get the fanciest cold press juicer on the market and rarely or inconsistently use it because it takes too much time. So what's the best juicer? It's the one you'll use every day.

Here are a few tips for purchasing a juicer:

Make sure your juicer is proficient at extracting the juice. Machines with overly high rpms can leave juice in the pulp. If you can squeeze juice out of the pulp, I wouldn't recommend that machine. Over the years, I have tried various juicers that are not capable of releasing all the juice, as they produce wet pulp. An inefficient juicer can be one reason why people end up spending a lot of money on produce. So you may save money in the long run by spending more up front on a good juicer.

Choose a strong machine that can juice all types of produce, including tough, hard items like broccoli stems, root vegetables like carrots and beets, and delicate foods like leafy greens and herbs. The masticating juicer will be the ticket if you do a lot of leafy greens, delicate herbs, or wheatgrass. Because they operate with a single or a double auger, they work well for pressing juice and processing leafy greens and herbs.

A large feed tube is a nice feature. Then you don't have to cut everything up in small pieces. A juicer with a large feed tube will save you time. Almost all the centrifugal juicers I've seen have a large opening for produce.

Make sure the machine ejects the pulp into a separate receptacle. Some of the older machines collect the pulp on the inside of the juice basket and the user must stop frequently to remove it. There are very few models like this anymore. But if you're at a garage sale or thrift store, which is about the only place you'll find one of them today, I'd recommend you pass it by. I have also seen one or two very cheap models that keep the pulp inside on sale at discount stores. Don't buy them.

Easy cleaning tip: Line the pulp receptacle with a plastic produce bag—one of the free baggies from the grocery store. By doing this, you can skip cleaning the container and simply plop the pulp into the trash or compost pile, or use it in cooking.

Simplify your life; cleaning and reassembling should be quick and simple. You don't want any extra work to keep you from daily juicing. If you buy a juicer with too many parts to clean, or the parts are complicated to wash, you probably won't juice every day. Also, make sure the parts are dishwasher safe. My routine is to rinse the juicer after use and leave it to air-dry. The blade basket is easy to clean, especially if you use the sink spray and a dish brush. It takes me only about a minute to clean all three parts (plus the plunger) of my juicer. Then occasionally I run the parts through the dishwasher to brighten everything up. Don't put the plunger in the dishwasher, though. I did this once and it swelled up with water to the point that I couldn't use it.

What about the Vitamix and NutriBullet blender types?

I am continually asked about the difference between juicers and blenders. Quite a few people think the blender they purchased is a juicer. They ask, "So what about the Magic Bullet? NutriBullet? Blendtec? Vitamix?" These are all blenders that keep everything in the container. They make smoothies, but not juice. Now, I love my Vitamix. I use it nearly every day to make my morning green smoothie. It's a wonderful addition to a healthy kitchen. I first make juice, pour that in my Vitamix, add an avocado, and blend until creamy. I put chopped almonds on top, and that's my breakfast— with a glass of juice.

Let's start with an explanation of the difference between a juicer and a blender. Many people are told to get one of the blender types because they should keep all the fiber. But I need to explain why this isn't very appetizing for many recipes made with vegetables. When you juice, you separate out the insoluble fiber or pulp from the juice. However, a blender simply blends up everything, leaving the insoluble fiber in the drink. I experimented with this by blending carrots, beet, parsley, and celery. The taste reminded me of fiber-thick mush. Lots of people say they end up straining their blended concoctions to get a palatable juice. But that takes *a lot* of time.

If you want the health benefits of juicing without giving up on taste and texture, you need a juicer, not a blender. When you blend up more fruit with leafy greens, you will get a tasty smoothie. But I've had many people say that to make it palatable, they had to use too much fruit and ended up with too much sugar. You could try what I do by juicing some of the veggies first and then pouring some in a blender and adding an avocado. For green smoothies with berries and other low-sugar fruit, see chapter 8. I have a number of smoothie recipes that don't require you to juice anything first. For your morning smoothies, you can use your Vitamix, NutriBullet, or other fast blender.

How do I get the best results from juicing?

The first step is no surprise: wash your produce.

Water seems to be quite effective against some external pesticides if you rinse the produce under running water for at least thirty seconds. Scientists at an experimental station in Connecticut washed produce with running water and discovered that it reduced pesticide residues for nine of twelve tested pesticides. It is interesting to note that some of the pesticides removed weren't even water-soluble, so they weren't dissolved in water but rather "mechanically pushed off the produce by the force of running water."[2]

If you prefer something stronger than water, many grocery stores and health food stores carry fruit and vegetable washes. Or you can make your own produce wash with baking soda and vinegar. Here is the formula for the baking soda wash: Mix several tablespoons of baking soda in a measuring cup with water and vinegar. Stir until dissolved and then pour into your sink of water. Use a vegetable brush to clean hard veggies and fruit. Then rinse. A vinegar-and-water solution destroys bacteria and mold. It's my first choice. Mix one cup white vinegar in a sink of water. Soak veggies and fruit in the solution. Scrub hard veggies and fruit with a veggie brush. Then rinse produce.

Washing your produce will get rid of surface pesticides and debris, but it will not pull out systemic pesticides—those in the water of the plant and fiber. That's why it is best to purchase organic produce, at least for the items on the Dirty Dozen list. (See more information later in this chapter.)

Cut away any moldy, bruised, or dinged areas of your produce.

You can't juice the peels of oranges, tangerines, tangelos, and grapefruit; they need to be peeled before juicing. Volatile oils are found in the skins of citrus fruit (except for lemons and limes) and can cause digestive problems. Organic lemon and lime peels can be juiced, but keep in mind that the flavor is quite distinct. Give it a try and see what you think. For some, it is not a favorite flavor in most recipes. I usually buy conventionally grown lemons and limes because they are closer to the Clean Fifteen. I peel them if they are not organic. Keep as much of the white pith from the peel as possible. It is here that you find the highest content of the vitamin C and bioflavonoids. These two nutrients interact with each other to create the best uptake for your cells. Also, peel mangoes and papayas. A harmful irritant is found in their skin, and you should not eat it, especially in quantity.

If you don't buy organic produce, my recommendation is to always peel your produce because the largest concentration of pesticides is found in the peel.

You see, two additives are often found on nonorganic produce: pesticides and wax. A nonorganic cucumber is an example of a vegetable that is waxed, and this wax traps the pesticides underneath. Neither pesticides nor wax should be in your juice.

5. Organic produce has better storability. Several studies of storability have shown that organic produce stores better than its counterpart and has a longer shelf life. This appears to be linked to lower nitrates in the produce.[13]

6. Organic produce tastes better. Better flavor appears to be linked to lower levels of nitrates in the food. For example, organic apples are generally preferred over those that are conventionally grown because of their flavor. Studies of organic apples' storability have been conducted in six different countries, where findings indicated they were "firmer and crisper when coming out of storage, and tend to hold more of their flavor."[14] Also, according to the Organic Center, a California study found that organic strawberries were sweeter and better looking.

AVOID THE DIRTY DOZEN

If you have a limited budget and can't afford to purchase all organic produce, at least avoid what the EWG calls the "Dirty Dozen." Each year this group prepares a report that shows the most heavily sprayed produce to the least heavily sprayed. You can also get an app for your phone to use when you shop to make sure you steer clear of the worst offenders. By just avoiding the top twelve most heavily sprayed produce items, it is estimated that you can reduce your pesticide exposure by 90 percent.[15] That is well worth the little extra money you might spend. But be encouraged—prices are coming down because more and more people want clean food, a.k.a. organic. The Dirty Dozen list changes each year. To get the current ratings, go to www.ewg.org.

The Dirty Dozen List

Here is the Dirty Dozen List as of 2017:[16]

- Strawberries
- Spinach
- Nectarines
- Apples
- Peaches
- Pears
- Cherries
- Grapes
- Celery
- Tomatoes
- Sweet bell peppers
- Potatoes

The Clean Fifteen List

The produce EWG lists as its "Clean Fifteen" has the least amount of pesticide spray residues, meaning these foods are the safest to consume as conventional produce.

As of 2017, the list includes the following:[17]

- Sweet corn
- Avocados
- Pineapples
- Cabbage
- Onions
- Sweet peas (frozen)
- Papayas
- Asparagus
- Mangoes
- Eggplant
- Honeydew melon
- Kiwi
- Cantaloupe
- Cauliflower
- Grapefruit

ARE MEXICAN IMPORTED ORGANICS TO BE TRUSTED?

It's winter and you're buzzing around the organic produce aisles. Half of what you want has a sticker that says it's from Mexico. Local options aren't available in most areas of the country in winter and early spring. But that Mexican sticker on your local grocery store produce can shoot up a "red, green, and white flag" question for some of us. How can we know that these veggies and fruits are reliable and safe for us to eat? Well, the most important thing to remember is this: "Organic imports from Mexico must meet USDA organic standards."[18]

Mexico has about fifteen certification agencies: "The National Organic Program (NOP) has been recognized and enforced since October 2002, when the United States implemented the Organic Food Production Act. In February 2006, the Mexican government published its own Law of Organic Products and with similar regulations. On-farm audits and regular border inspections are important parts of organic certification and food safety testing in Mexico."[19]

It's estimated that Mexico has more than 110,000 organic farmers, with more than 90 percent farming on less than nine acres. When you buy Mexican organics, you support a proud group of organic Mexican farmers who take great pride in producing their food. Organic farming allows them to remain on their land and be part of their community rather than having to move to a big city to find work.[20]

THE DANGERS OF IRRADIATED FOOD

If you have never seen food irradiated, you probably don't even think about this practice when you go to the grocery store. But it's a process that is happening often. Irradiation exposes food, including fruits and vegetables, to ionizing radiation to destroy microorganisms, bacteria, viruses, or insects. Food producers rely on gamma radiation to kill off the unwanted microorganisms and to extend shelf life. But at what cost? The fruits and vegetables still look OK, but what happens to the nutrients is the reason to stay away. Irradiation destroys vitamins, enzymes, phytonutrients, and biophotons. It also produces harmful free radicals that damage cells along with a harmful radiolytic by-product known as thalidomide.

Dr. George Tritsch of Roswell Park Memorial Institute, New York State Department of Health, has opposed irradiated food "because of the abundant and convincing evidence in the refereed scientific literature that the condensation products of the free radicals formed during irradiation produce statistically significant increases in carcinogenesis, mutagenesis and cardiovascular disease in animals and man."[21]

There is one more reason to avoid irradiated foods. Irradiating fruits and vegetables causes even greater problems than irradiating other foods because they have a large water content. This creates the perfect environment for formation of more free radicals—those toxic molecules that damage our cells. Irradiation is not the answer. Rather, it lies in not overusing pesticides, which creates weak plants, and in sustainable farming. To make sure you avoid irradiated produce, buy organic.

JUMP OFF THE GMO FOOD TRAIN

In 2016, Jeffrey Smith, founder of the Institute for Responsible Technology, received the much-deserved Lifetime Achievement Award from The Truth About Cancer for his tireless work in exposing the dangers of genetically modified foods.[22] "There is more than a casual association between GM foods and adverse health effects," Smith says. "'There is causation,' as defined by recognized scientific criteria. 'The strength of association and consistency between GM foods and disease is confirmed in several animal studies.'"[23]

Depending on the research, you will read conflicting results. It seems it all depends on who funded the studies. For a clearer picture, you may want to read the 2010 book *The World According to Monsanto*, by Marie-Monique Robin.

There are at least twelve good reasons to avoid genetically modified foods:[24]

1. Try organ damage, for a starter. According to animal studies, GMOs also affect the gastrointestinal tract and the immune system. And have you ever wondered why so many young women have trouble getting pregnant these days? GMOs can cause infertility. And it can

even accelerate the aging process. Monsanto researchers studied three strains of GM maize (corn) fed to animals and they showed signs of liver and kidney damage. Of these strains, two of them were genetically modified to synthesize insecticide toxins, and the third was manipulated to resist herbicides.[25] These three strains of GMO corn are grown for humans to eat in America. Reports show that Monsanto released this information only after a legal challenge from Greenpeace and other groups against GMO foods.[26]

2. These genetically modified plants can contaminate the earth forever. GMO plants have been shown to be so insidious that they can even outlast nuclear waste.

3. GMOs increase herbicide use. "Between 1996 and 2008, US farmers sprayed an extra 383 million pounds of herbicide on GMOs. Overuse of Roundup results in 'superweeds' resistant to the herbicide. This is causing farmers to use even more toxic herbicides every year. Not only does this create environmental harm, GM foods contain higher residues of toxic herbicides. Roundup, for example, is linked with sterility, hormone disruption, birth defects, and cancer."[27]

4. GMOs can produce "new toxins, allergens, carcinogens, and nutritional deficiencies."[28]

5. GMOs destroy life on this planet. They can hurt wildlife and even soil organisms. Are you wondering what has happened to the monarch butterfly population? Researchers believe GMOs have contributed to their demise.

6. Are you tired of chemicals flooding our earth? GMOs require large amounts of chemicals to grow, which are harmful to our air, soil, and water.

7. There is an epidemic of superweed crops that are attributed to GMOs. We now have superweeds that have taken over some farm areas; they are even resistant to the chemicals used on GMO crops.

8. For all the discourse on greenhouse gas, have you ever heard that 50 percent of the total emissions of nitrous oxide is attributed to GMO crops?

9. Do you want to protect our organic produce? Speak out. GMO crops contaminate these crops.

10. GMOs damage our ecosystem and the beneficial insects.

11. GMO companies control the seed industry and our food supply. Farmers are forced to buy new seed each year because many crops don't produce seeds that can be planted.

12. Farmers are not allowed to save their seeds from crops that do have reproducible seeds due to the "police efforts" of big agri-biz companies.

SHOP SMART

Become a smart shopper and avoid GMOs. To do this, you need to be very cognizant of the top genetically engineered crops, which are soybeans and corn. To date, it is not mandatory to label products GMOs. The big companies have effectively beat down all legislative attempts at GMO labeling in state after state. Some experts estimate that up to thirty thousand different products on grocery store shelves are genetically modified because a good percentage of that number of foods contain soy. About 90 percent of our soy crop in America is GMO.[29] To obtain a GMO shopping guide, go to http://responsibletechnology.org/10-reasons-to-avoid-gmos/.

CHAPTER 5

CHOOSING YOUR
BEST MOVES

ADEQUATE EXERCISE PLUS proper diet is an equation for success. Sipping Skinny drinks and a low-carb diet plan combined with physical activity will propel you into a slim, toned, and energetic body.

A sedentary lifestyle has become commonplace in today's society. Our bodies are designed to be active but have slipped into stillness (or should I say "stiffness"?) through years of inactivity. Many of us pass most of our time sitting behind desks or submerged in high-stress environments that leave us feeling drained. The gift of movement has become the work of exercise—hence we call it a "workout." Along with the pressures of our fast-paced lives, we often consume foods that lack nutritious value and hinder our ability to feel alive and energized. We often reach for taste-good snacks at the end of a stressful day that lack anything close to nutrition.

On the bright side, you can make major changes with a minimal amount of consistent exercise. Your muscles will feel nourished and strong, and you will radiate health and beauty throughout your entire being.

The benefits of exercise are abundant. Muscles, bones, and connective tissues are strengthened with exercise. A fitness regimen creates a physique that is resilient and fit. Not only is it advantageous to your outward appearance, but most importantly, movement creates a multitude of benefits for the internal organs. Exercise builds new proteins and hormones, keeps the heart and cardiovascular system healthy, strengthens the immune system, boosts growth hormones that help build muscles, enables nutrients to metabolize, carries waste products out of our systems, relieves stress, promotes peaceful sleep, and burns calories.

Our quality of sleep is also improved by proper exercise. When we lack quality sleep, we tend to crave unhealthy foods, especially carbohydrates. Also, appetite-stimulating hormones will spike, causing us to eat more than usual.

Almost any health-care professional will reaffirm the importance of exercise to lose weight and feel great. You can start off small and gradually increase your exercise. Your rewards are better health and weight loss. If you haven't exercised before or haven't done much working out in a while, begin with just thirty minutes of moderate exercise, such as a brisk walk. Even this minimal amount will facilitate physical fitness and weight loss.

IMPROVE YOUR HORMONES WITH EXERCISE

Weight is directly affected by about eight hormones, which will improve with exercise.

Insulin

The pancreas produces insulin, a peptide hormone that regulates fat metabolism and carbohydrates. To promote the absorption and storage of glucose and glycogen, insulin is released when blood sugar is elevated. Glucose levels in the blood are reduced by insulin, therefore aiding and promoting absorption from fat tissues or skeletal muscles to the bloodstream. It is significant to understand that instead of being used to propel muscle activity, insulin can cause fat to accumulate in adipose tissue. Physical activity causes the suppression of insulin in the sympathetic nervous system. Avoiding high-sugar foods, especially before exercise (sports drinks included), is necessary, because they cause insulin levels to elevate and glycogen to be stored instead of being burned for fuel. (I recommend you avoid high-sugar foods at all times.)

Glucagon

Manufactured by the pancreas, glucagon is released in reaction to low levels of blood sugar. Its objective is to stimulate free fatty acids (FFAs) from adipose tissue and accelerate adequate blood glucose levels. These are both equally important for sustaining activity. As exercise depletes levels of glycogen, glucagon releases additional glycogen that the liver has stored.

Cortisol

Created by the adrenal glands, cortisol is a catabolic steroid hormone that responds to exercise, low blood sugar, and stress. During prolonged periods of working out, cortisol supports energy metabolism. It assists in the breakdown of protein and triglycerides, creating the necessary glucose to aid in sustaining exercise. When the body does not fully recover from a previous workout and experiences an overabundance of physical stress, cortisol is released. Cortisol also helps with metabolizing fat. But when we have too much cortisol, often pumped out in response to stress, it can be responsible for depositing fat, especially on the midsection.

Norepinephrine and epinephrine

The sympathetic nervous system (SNS) is dramatically assisted by these amine hormones. They play a starring role in regulating the body's function during cardio exercise and also produce energy. Even though norepinephrine and epinephrine are related hormones, they perform separately. Adrenaline is the common name for epinephrine because it is produced by the adrenal glands. It increases blood sugar to help fuel exercise, elevates cardiac output, supports fat metabolism, and encourages the breakdown of glycogen for energy. Norepinephrine has all of these functions in common with epinephrine; in addition, it constricts blood vessels in body parts that are not being exercised.

Testosterone

Leydig cells of male testes and ovaries in females produce a steroid hormone called testosterone. Both genders also produce trace amounts in the adrenal glands. When muscle proteins are damaged by exercise, testosterone is in charge of repair and muscle protein resynthesis. Testosterone also significantly assists the growth of skeletal muscle. It is produced in response to damaged muscle proteins and works with specific receptor sites.

Human growth hormone

Cellular growth is stimulated by an anabolic peptide hormone called human growth hormone (HGH). It is secreted by the anterior pituitary gland. While working with specific receptor sites, HGH can produce responses such as increased bone materialization, muscle protein synthesis and lipolysis, elevated immune system function, and metabolized fat. During rapid eye movement (REM) sleep cycles, HGH is created in the body. This hormone is stimulated by strength training or high intensity cardio exercise.

Insulin-like growth factor

The same mechanisms that manufacture HGH are stimulated by insulin-like growth factor (IGF), which is similar to insulin in molecular structure. When it comes to improving muscle growth, IGF is a valuable hormone. The number of calories burned at a resting heart rate depends on the amount of muscle you have. The liver produces this peptide hormone, which repairs damaged proteins due to exercise. It also assists in the function of HGH.

Brain-derived neurotrophic factor

The production of new cells in the brain is stimulated by a neurotransmitter referred to as brain-derived neurotrophic factor (BDNF). The generation of BDNF, HGH, and IGF are all closely related. The levels of these hormones are elevated by the same exercises. Anabolic hormones, which contribute to muscle growth, are accelerated by high-intensity exercise. Levels of BDNF become elevated, which can enhance cognitive function.

Wow! Are you impressed that you get to kick all this into action when you work out? I never knew just how important exercise was to a health body until I began studying the hormones connected with exercise.

EXERCISE THAT MAKES A DIFFERENCE

Exercise helps you to feel amazing while you're dropping those extra pounds. There are a multitude of diverse ways to get active. While you may already have a fitness routine, perhaps this chapter will inspire you to try out something new. It is fun and exciting to diversify a workout. Specific movements are geared toward different results. Here are some suggestions that are divided up into three broad categories: aerobic exercises, weight and resistance training, and strengthening and stretching exercises. Choosing something from each category will result in a balanced routine. Exercising forty-five to sixty minutes, three to four times a week, is an excellent initial goal. Consistency is the most crucial factor. Keep up with your program, and you will be happy with the results. If you have trouble staying motivated, you may want to get a personal trainer or join some exercise classes.

Aerobic exercise

The definition of *aerobic* is "in the presence of oxygen." In order to produce energy, each cell in the body requires oxygen. Maximum energy is brought into our cells through aerobic activities. These are sustained activities that depend on oxygen for energy. These activities burn fat, condition the cardiovascular system, and build endurance.

You can start your exercise program with thirty to forty minutes of workouts, three to four times per week, especially if you are a beginner or have been inactive for a while. It is best to increase the time and intensity of your workout as you gain strength and progress in your exercise regimen. Choose from the various activities that are emphasized in this chapter (or maybe something not mentioned). Remember that the greatest benefits come from consistency.

Go at your own pace and listen to your body. If you have any health concerns, check with a doctor and then get active.

Sitting down for extended periods or living a high-stress lifestyle builds up excess emotional energy and chemicals in the body that will dissipate through aerobic exercise. Taking a break to exercise can alleviate unhealthy actions such as drinking large amounts of coffee, eating too much food, taking drugs, or lashing out at coworkers, spouses, or kids. Working out dispels pent-up emotions and channels them into a positive outlet.

There are many enjoyable aerobic activities that are also effective for weight loss, such as dancing, bicycling, walking, swimming, jogging, skiing, or racquet sports. Remember the days when step aerobics was the craze? Now not too many health clubs offer step classes. Check out your local club to see what they offer. Find something you love to do. It is a lot easier to stick with it when you're having fun.

The following pages contain some options to choose from. There is also an abundance of creative activities that are not listed here. So get creative. Just remember to keep moving a little bit more each week. Even small changes, like taking the stairs instead of an elevator or parking your car further away from the entrance, can add up. Activity will rev up your metabolism, and you will begin to burn more calories. This even holds true at a resting heart rate. Your muscles will strengthen, and you will look more toned and feel more energized as you generate a higher degree of weight loss.

High-intensity intermittent exercise (HIIE) for fat loss

What is HIIE? Quite simply, it is a form of high-intensity intermittent exercise that alternates short periods of intense anaerobic exercise with less intense recovery periods. According to *Women's Health* magazine, some of the benefits are that it strengthens the heart muscle, represents the fitness equivalent of a "buy one get one free" offer, doesn't require a gym, and keeps your blood sugar in check.[1]

Studies show that this type of exercise increases aerobic and anaerobic fitness: "HIIE also significantly lowers insulin resistance and results in a number of skeletal muscle adaptations that result in enhanced skeletal muscle fat oxidation and improved glucose tolerance."[2]

How do you engage in this kind of exercise? Many clubs offer this type of activity. It's probably best to have some guidance to know just what you should do. But if you're adventuresome, you may be able to set up a plan for yourself by simply reading about it on the web.

Bicycling—a.k.a. cycling

Though it is a low-impact activity, when done for a sufficient length of time and with high intensity, cycling is an excellent aerobic conditioner. You will not raise your heart rate merely by coasting around the neighborhood on a bicycle. However, sustained cycling will increase endurance, reduce stress, and build strength in the back and legs. It is capable of burning up to 350–450 calories an hour, depending on the speed and terrain.

Running can be stressful on the body, which makes cycling popular due to its low impact. People who have orthopedic problems, conditions aggravated by weight-bearing exercises, or are overweight find cycling to be an excellent choice.

When the weather is not great, outdoor biking may not be the most desirable choice. Ah, the indoor stationary bike to the rescue! It is a viable alternative that will keep bike enthusiasts just as fit. Most people have more motivation when working out with a group, which is one reason cycling classes are popular at most health clubs.

Did you ever think that cycling could make you smarter? Check out the research that includes this statement: "Cycling gets the nerve cells in your brain firing and as these neurons spark into action they foster the production of proteins such as brain-derived neurotrophic factor (BDNF). It also helps your neurotransmitters communicate more effectively."[3] So as you're pedaling away in the fresh air or your own home, you can be improving your memory and concentration.

Adequate movement is necessary for the lymphatic system to properly excrete toxic wastes. Physical exercise or lymphatic drainage massage is required to move lymph through the body. And since lymph is a big carrier of waste, moving it along is important to the detoxification of the body. Waste is assisted out of the body very successfully by rebounding, which increases lymph flow fifteen to thirty times its normal rate. We often will feel tired and sick when we lack adequate exercise to move the lymph. A lack of exercise may also contribute to depression, a general sense of malaise, headache, and aching muscles. This is a toxic state that will eventually lead to many degenerative diseases, such as arthritis, heart disease, cancer, and even premature aging.

There are many health-enhancing benefits that come from rebounding. It promotes deep relaxation, improves weight loss, and helps build muscle. Metabolic rate is also improved, so even after exercising, more calories continue to burn. In addition, oxygen is circulated to the tissues, where it is greatly needed. The heart and other muscles in the body work more efficiently as they are strengthened by rebounding. It improves digestion and elimination while lowering triglycerides and cholesterol.

Bouncing slowly is the best way to begin rebounding. Your body moves up and down while your feet keep in contact with the rebounder's surface. Oxygen will begin to move through your torso, limbs, and into your head after only a few minutes.

Your entire body will strengthen with this movement. You can begin to bounce faster and higher as your balance and strength increase. Turn on music, watch television, or even talk on the phone—rebounding allows you to do other things while you bounce.

Running shoes may be worn, or just jump in your bare feet. But don't wear just socks, because they can be slippery. Five to ten minutes is a good starting point; gradually increase your time as you become more fit. A few minutes several times a day will work well if you are out of shape or older; you can steadily build up your time. Prolapsed organs are the only contraindication to rebounding. If you have this condition, you could start with just a few minutes and build up, provided your doctor gives the OK. The connective tissues around the internal organs will then have time to strengthen.

For someone with physical limitations, the rebounder is ideal. Rebounding provides freedom to exercise for those who have knee or joint problems. There is even a hand rail that can be attached to the rebounder for handicapped or blind people. Children who are hyperactive have even been reported to calm down after only a few days of bouncing.

Lymphasizer (swing machine): an exercise machine for everyone

Designed by a Japanese doctor, the lymphasizer is a terrific addition or ideal alternative to an exercise regimen. When you lie down on the floor with your feet on the machine, it actively moves the blood and lymph through your body. People with circulation problems in the feet that stem from steroid drug use or diabetes can benefit from its gentle rocking action. This machine requires no active movement and results in a zero-impact workout. In about ten to fifteen minutes you can obtain benefits similar to a thirty-minute aerobic exercise by just lying on the floor with your feet in the grooves.

This machine is perfect for you if you have a physical limitation. There is absolutely no stress applied to the knees, ankles, or other body parts when engaging in this simple exercise. The lymphasizer will rock your body from side to side as you simply lie there. It moves the body in a motion similar to that of a swimming fish. A good oxygen supply and energy balance is maintained. Stress reduction and relaxation are achieved with regular use of this relaxing movement. You will immediately notice that this massaging swing action creates a sense of well-being. Restful sleep and even weight loss are promoted by using this machine.

For people who are unable to bounce slowly on the rebounder because they are disabled or have medical issues, the lymphasizer is very useful. It is also excellent for those who are very overweight, have serious ankle or knee problems, or just find other forms of exercise very difficult. (See the Resources section at the end of the book for more information on the lymphasizer.)

Step and dance aerobics

Many people prefer to work out in a class setting because it is motivating, pushes them to try harder, and is fun. It also has a set schedule and membership fee, which helps hold you accountable. Also, you can make new friends who have similar goals. It reinforces your personal commitment without having to rely entirely on yourself to get off the couch and get motivated. There are a large variety of classes at most gyms and health clubs. Options include dance aerobics, step aerobics, non-step aerobics, and total body workout classes that involve the use of light weights with lots of aerobic movement. Experiment with different classes and have fun! One of my favorites is the total body workout.

Swimming

An excellent cardiovascular workout that tones the entire body, swimming improves the delivery of oxygen to muscles and strengthens your heart. This is one of the top sports to stimulate circulation and build muscle while putting zero stress on the joints. It regulates breathing and soothes the mind. Swimming is ideal for almost everyone—the overweight; young; old; people with ankle, knee and joint problems; and people who are healthy and in shape. Swimming is even great for weight loss because it has a calorie-burning potential of 350–420 calories per hour.

Water aerobics

A variety of techniques from land aerobics are usually combined into water aerobic workouts. These exercises include jumping jacks, running forward and backward, walking with various arm movements, or mimicking cross-country skiing. There is also special equipment that may be incorporated such as wrist and ankle weights, water aerobics shoes for walking around the pool, flotation devices, and belts. Music may be used, or the exercises can be done in silence.

Being in the water reduces the risk of muscle or joint injury and supports the body. A greater range of motion is achieved by floatation because it decreases gravity and places less stress on the joints when stretching. Water aerobics is especially safe for the elderly because of the easing of gravity. The body is also continuously cooled while exercising in the water, thus preventing overheating. The duration of a basic water aerobics class is about forty-five to sixty minutes.

Zumba dance

A Zumba routine resembles a dance party more than it does a workout. It is a one-of-a-kind fitness program that incorporates easy-to-follow moves with Latin rhythms. Zumba participants engage in exciting, energizing dance movements. You will burn calories while having an absolute blast. Interval training sessions are featured in the routines where resistance training and slow and fast rhythms are combined to burn fat while sculpting and toning the body. Add some international music into the mix, spiced up with a lot of Latin flavor, and it's time to Zumba! Go to a local club and check out a class. This is definitely an excellent workout! I took a class and danced so hard I was dripping sweat and sporting a giant smile on my face by the time it was over.

Walking

Practically everyone is capable of walking. You can fast walk or stroll for exercise anywhere, and calories will burn along the way. You can even walk indoors. To keep in the midrange of aerobic activity, walk at a brisk pace. This will keep strain off your ligaments and joints, unlike some other more vigorous forms of aerobic activity.

Your sense of well-being increases while walking, as it does with most forms of movement. Some of the advantages of walking include mood elevation, lessened symptoms of anxiety and depression, relaxation of tight muscles, and reduced stress. It will also help you sleep better when you walk in the evening after dinner. Getting out in the fresh air may be part of the key.

A consistent walking program may include some of the following:

- Walk without losing your breath, but fast enough to break a sweat. In order to regain a resting heart rate, slow down toward the end of your walk.

- Enjoy a brisk walk before or after dinner. It will burn calories while relaxing your nervous system.

- Walking with a friend provides motivation and companionship. Dogs are excellent walking partners as well. Maybe you can walk the neighbor's dog if you don't have one of your own. You will be drawn to the simpler things in life and be inspired to keep moving with your canine companion by your side. I will contest to that! In addition to my exercise classes two to four times a week, I walk Annie Mae. Since I started, my thighs have become considerably firmer.

Weight and resistance training

One of the most efficient ways to develop muscle tone and strength is by doing weight-bearing exercises, such as strength training with machines, or by using free weights. Lean body mass increases with this form of exercise, which is important for facilitating weight loss. The body is forced to produce more muscle when weight training. Mitochondria are cell organelles that produce energy and burn glucose. High concentrations of them are found in skeletal and heart muscles. This is where nutrients from the food we eat are burned to produce adenosine triphosphate (ATP), which in turn produces cellular energy—thus, mitochondria are referred to as cellular furnaces. (The major source of energy for cellular reactions is ATP, a nucleotide derived from adenosine that occurs in muscle tissue.)

The connective tissues and bones are also strengthened by weight and resistance training. This aids in the prevention of injuries and osteoporosis. Balance and coordination are also improved when one performs this type of exercise.

Weight training or resistance training increases endurance and strengthens, tones, and builds muscles. After only a few short weeks of a concentrated weight training program, you will begin to look leaner and more toned.

The body has a natural tendency to grow weaker with age, but weight training will counteract this process. Weight-bearing exercise is an essential component of osteoporosis prevention. After the age of twenty-five, we can lose up to half a pound of muscle every year unless we include regular strength training. You will look leaner and more toned and stay stronger longer if you include weight training. Gyms with weight training programs often have men and women in their sixties and seventies (and even eighties) who resemble fit and trim fifty-year-olds. This may inspire and encourage you to incorporate some form of strength training into your regular routine.

No matter how weak, old, or out of shape you are or think you are, it is still possible to improve your appearance, boost your strength, and lose weight.

Strengthening and stretching exercises

Exercises that relax the mind while strengthening and stretching the body have been used throughout history. The preeminent goal is to relax and stretch the muscles while controlling the breath. This delivers more oxygen into the cells, especially the brain cells, therefore relaxing and calming the entire body.

Breathing and stretching exercises can enhance physical and mental relaxation, improve your quality of sleep, and increase suppleness. No matter what level of ability you have or what age you are, stretching is available to us all. Ideal methods of relaxation include deep breathing, long stretches, and gentle movements. This is recommended as the best type of exercise to engage in toward the end of the day so that the body does not get overstimulated and is more at ease. For those who only have time to exercise in the evening, these techniques are an outstanding choice, because strenuous exercise can be overstimulating and could keep you awake.

One of the advantages of stretching is that it relieves anxiety and stress because it strengthens the nervous system. It also relaxes and strengthens the muscular, cardiovascular, skeletal, glandular, digestive, and nervous systems while contributing to a calm mind and body.

Toning combo workout classes

My favorite classes at my club are "Peak Physique" and "Ballet Bootcamp." The first is a combination of stretching, sit-ups, balls, balance, and hand weights. The bootcamp offers a workout at the barre along with sit-ups, hand weights, and stretching.

Pilates

Strength and flexibility are improved through Pilates, a series of balancing and stretching exercises that give people a leaner, longer appearance. This exercise series was created by a prisoner of war during World War II named Joseph Pilates. It has risen in popularity in recent years. While in a German internment camp, Pilates demonstrated his exercises to fellow inmates to help them stay physically and mentally fit. He also introduced the mat workout.

The Pilates exercise series is particularly popular among athletes, models, dancers, and celebrities. It helps improve posture and develop flexibility without putting any strain on the joints. A continuous Pilates regimen will increase mobility in joints, flatten the stomach, slim the thighs, and sculpt the waist. The body will be less prone to injury while practicing Pilates. It will also improve flexibility, balance, tone, and strength. The deep Pilates stretching boosts energy, relieves tension, and reduces stress. The spine and back are also strengthened. People seeking rehabilitation after injuries to their limbs are encouraged to engage in Pilates. It is recommended for everyone—the elderly, young, overweight, those who suffer from osteoporosis, and people who have been living a sedentary lifestyle.

Yoga stretch

Yoga is a low-impact ancient art. When it is continuously practiced, a sense of well-being spreads throughout the body and mind, creating clarity and emotional stability. If you shy away from the spiritual aspect of yoga, there are classes that focus on the physical side. Practicing yoga strengthens the body and increases flexibility. It improves the circulatory, hormonal, respiratory, and digestive systems. An instructor will help you to gain proper alignment, thus rebalancing your body. This induces a greater flow of energy and aids in decreasing health problems. There are also gentler forms of yoga that are well suited for beginners and the elderly. Most studios offer a wide range of classes, or you can just start with some videos at home. Experiment with the different styles and discover which ones resonate with you. Check out yoga stretches you can do every day.[6]

YOUR SKINNY SKIPPING
EXERCISE SCHEDULE

There is an amazing adventure awaiting in the vast world of exercise. Research continues to prove the outstanding benefits of exercise. A recent study conducted by researchers at Duke University Medical Center demonstrated the impact that six months of exercise had on fifty-three participants with sedentary lifestyles. Four levels of activity were measured—the equivalents of twelve miles of jogging per week, twelve miles of walking per week, twenty miles of jogging per week, and inactivity. The participants exercised on elliptical trainers, treadmills, or cycle ergometers. Benefits were displayed after even a moderate amount of exercise.[7]

Pick at least three days a week to exercise for at least an hour. Plan what you will do and stick to it. Classes at a gym are nice because there's a set time when you have to be there. You also have other people to interact with and spur you on.

Now write down what you are going to do for the week, and don't waver. Treat this as if it were a job. You can exercise more than three times a week but not less. I'm giving you a three-day plan here to choose what you want to do. Fill in the blanks with your activity or class, the day of the week you will start, and the time of day.

Here's your plan:

DAY 1

Activity: _____

Day of the week: _____

Time: _____

DAY 2

Activity: _____

Day of the week: _____

Time: _____

DAY 3

Activity: _____

Day of the week: _____

Time: _____

GRAB YOUR WORKOUT SHOES AND GO FOR IT!

Now is the time to set your mind to "just do it!" Stay consistent and reap the many rewards of a healthy active lifestyle. It doesn't take much to make a significant difference so you can look and feel fabulous inside and out.

CHAPTER 6

WHEN WEIGHT LOSS PLATEAUS HAPPEN TO GOOD PEOPLE

S O HERE YOU are, skipping along on your Sipping Skinny program, losing weight each week. Then one day you get on the scale and it hasn't budged. You pick it up and tap it a few times. Try again. Nope. It's stuck where it was last week. You give it a good hard shake. That'll do it. No luck. It's still in the same place. What happened?

If you suddenly can't seem to move the scale down despite your best efforts, (a.k.a. a weight loss plateau), you may need an intervention that gets to the root of why you aren't losing the weight. Correct the issue, and you'll be back on your way to weight loss joy.

When weight loss comes to a standstill (and it can happen to the best of us), sometimes there's more to it than simply eating too many calories and not exercising enough. So take a deep breath. Back away from the scale. Take time to "check under the hood" to see what may be going on inside your body that is keeping you from shedding those unwanted pounds. Whatever you do, don't abandon the Sipping Skinny ship of juices, smoothies, and broths that have helped so many other people sail into weight loss glory. If your weight is hanging on like gum to the sole of your shoe, look up! This chapter is for you.

WHAT'S YOUR ISSUE?

"If I had an hour to solve a problem, I'd spend fifty-five minutes thinking about the problem and five minutes thinking about solutions." Though this quote is often attributed to Albert Einstein, some question whether the legendary inventor actually said it.[1] Nevertheless, this quote represents a helpful way to approach one's physical health. The bad news is that there are a number of problems (i.e., health conditions and lifestyle issues) that can inhibit weight loss. The good news is that once you take the time to identify your particular problem, you can address it and solve the weight loss resistance mystery.

Take heart. As Charlotte Gerson, daughter of the eminent Dr. Max Gerson, says, "You can't keep one disease and heal two others. When the body heals, it heals everything."[2] In the same way, you can't keep one symptom—like weight loss resistance—and heal two others when they are all caused by the same underlying condition or issue. When you get to the root of your particular health challenge and heal your body, all your related symptoms will fade away and weight loss can continue. Here's more good news: as you detoxify your organs through elimination, balance your hormones, identify and eliminate problematic foods that cause weight gain, and ultimately heal your body, you can achieve and maintain a healthy weight for life. It is possible.

As you review each condition in this chapter, consider if you have any other physical symptoms aside from weight loss resistance. Many people are unaware of symptoms that could suggest dysfunction in the body, especially if they are relatively minor, if they have come on gradually, and/or if they have become chronic issues (to the extent that one has accepted them as normal). It may be helpful to write down anything you experience on a regular basis that causes you discomfort or frustration, no matter how minor or unrelated your symptoms may seem. You may be surprised by what your body is trying to tell you.

IS YOUR LIVER HAPPY?

I've had a number of people come to me who hit a weight loss plateau. The first thing I recommend is a liver detox. The liver is the major fat metabolism organ in the body. When it is overloaded with toxins and waste, you won't lose weight.

So how do you know whether you have a happy, properly functioning liver or an unhappy, toxic one? If you tend to gain weight around your middle, if you have a potbelly that you just can't seem to get rid of, or if you find yourself with a "spare tire" around your upper abdomen, then your liver may not be regulating fat metabolism efficiently. It could even have an unhealthy excess of fatty tissue, a condition known as fatty liver. If you want to lose that stubborn abdominal fat, the liver must first be cleansed so that it can get back to burning fat efficiently. Once proper liver functions are restored, all that extra weight that refused to leave will begin to gradually melt away, often without much effort.

But let's get back to that term *fatty liver* for a second. When someone has a fatty liver, it means the liver has transformed from a spry, fat-metabolizing machine into a lazy fat-storage unit. You might wonder, "Why would my liver turn on me like that?" It's important to understand the liver is the body's main organ of detoxification. It filters and cleanses around fifty gallons of blood every day in order to remove toxins from the body and keep it healthy and functioning properly. But if the amount of toxins and rate at which they are introduced into the body are greater than the liver's ability to process them, then the liver will begin storing toxins in fat cells to protect the body from their damaging effects. And the more toxins the liver stores, the more fat it accumulates, the more the liver becomes congested, and the more liver functions are compromised, including fat metabolism. In short, it's a domino effect of health and weight loss complications.

The good news is that both liver toxicity and fatty liver can be reversed. Sipping Skinny is just the program to do that. It centers on juices, smoothies, and broths that contain a variety of the vegetables and fruits that make livers most happy. Raw vegetable and fruit smoothies in particular increase both soluble and insoluble fiber in the gut. This is essential to reducing the recirculation of unwanted fat and toxins back to the liver.

If you suspect you have a fatty liver, keep in mind that just as your liver gradually retained all its excess fat, so it will gradually lose the fat. But keep your eye on the prize, which is both improved health and significantly easier weight loss. As you Sip Skinny your juice, smoothie, or broth, it can be helpful to visualize it traveling through your digestive system, permeating your cells, healing everything it touches, and melting off a little more fat each time. In the end you'll be drinking away those pounds and restoring your body to health.

A note for menopausal women: In addition to toxins, the wrong type of hormone replacement therapy can overload the liver and prevent it from burning fat. This can lead to weight loss resistance and weight gain. If you are menopausal and overweight, consider hormone replacement therapy that bypasses the liver, such as hormone patches, creams, or buccal lozenges (troches).

Liver-happy foods

- Apples are a wonderful source of pectin, a soluble fiber that helps filter toxins out of the bloodstream. Apples also contain multiple phytochemicals that aid in detoxification.

- Avocados are extremely nourishing and packed with fiber, which helps protect the liver by preventing unhealthy fat and unwanted toxins from recirculating back to it.

- Broccoli, cauliflower, cabbage, and other cruciferous vegetables support the body's production of glutathione, a powerful antioxidant that assists the liver in removing toxins from the body.[3]

- Carrots and beets are full of flavonoids and beta-carotene, which improve liver function.

- Garlic (when consumed raw) is a significant source of allicin and selenium, which help to cleanse the liver.[4]

- Leafy green vegetables are rich in chlorophyll, which not only gives them their vibrant, green color but also binds to and removes toxins, helping to relieve the liver of its toxic load.

- Lemon juice activates the release of enzymes that help transform fat-soluble toxins into a water-soluble form so the body can flush them out.[5]

HAS TOXICITY HIJACKED YOUR WEIGHT LOSS?

To put it simply, a toxin is a foreign substance that does not belong in your body and causes it harm. Often the damaging effects of toxins are so insidious in undermining your health that you don't necessarily notice any problems right away. But it's only a matter of time until these substances take their toll on the body—substances like the chemicals used in pesticides on inorganically grown crops, plastics, nonstick cookware, cosmetics and personal care products, house cleaning solvents, dryer sheets, synthetic fragrances in everything from air fresheners to scented trash bags, and many other common products we use or are exposed to every day.

It's not unusual for people who struggle with weight loss to blame themselves for not having enough discipline or willpower. Forget that! Here's the deal: the more toxins we ingest or surround ourselves with on a regular basis, the more they break down the body's natural defenses and weight control mechanisms. Again, when the

may serve as a quick energy fix to get by in the moment, but it only continues the harmful cycle, and the insulin-resistant person is even worse off than before, not to mention carrying around more weight, again usually around one's midsection.

So, what to do, what to do? Unfortunately, today's standard American diet (aptly abbreviated as SAD) largely revolves around prepackaged foods that typically contain highly processed, nutrient-depleted carbohydrates. If you want to turn around insulin resistance, it starts with cutting out processed carbohydrates, especially refined sugar and flour. Sipping Skinny is the best way to heal the cellular and fat metabolism dysfunction that comes from insulin resistance. But you will want to adjust your juicing recipes to include only low-sugar fruits like green apples, berries, lemons, and limes.

Yes, this means eliminating sugar and even reducing fruit intake temporarily. What about natural sweeteners like honey, brown rice syrup, and pure maple syrup? While they do contain some nutrients and aren't bleached and refined, natural sweeteners are still sugar. If you want to say good-bye to insulin resistance, you need to restore your body's sensitivity to insulin by maintaining healthy and steady blood sugar levels which, for the time being, means saying good-bye to all sugar. Don't cry! It really does get easier each day. If I could do it, you can too. As you regain insulin sensitivity, weight loss should follow quite naturally. Eventually, you should be able to add a larger variety of fruit back into your diet, although you will still want to limit high-sugar fruit and always consume it with the fiber it naturally contains. In other words, rather than juicing higher-sugar fruit, either eat it whole or throw it in a smoothie with plenty of alkalizing greens.

BLOOD SUGAR DROP

On my Watercress Soup and Smoothie Diet, Shirley's blood sugar dropped from 200 to 141 in two days and then to normal in less than two weeks. She says, "I lost a total of four pounds and one inch off my waist. The amazing thing is the health benefits. My blood sugar is staying stable, my skin issues are clearing, and my face is more firm and elastic. I noticed this morning that my eyelashes are thicker and more brown. I don't have very thick eyelashes, so I was grateful for this result. I have less body stiffness, more energy, and sleep better. I wake up with a clearer head." Shirley isn't alone; Patricia's blood sugar dropped from 359 to 116 in about the same amount of time.

It may seem daunting to cut out sugar from your diet, and you may even be doubtful that your palate can ever grow accustomed to vegetable juices and smoothies without the help of high-sugar fruit like pineapple or bananas. But you will notice that as you Sip Skinny on a regular basis, your taste buds will change. In fact, your body will begin to crave fresh vegetable juices and smoothies as they feed your cells essential nutrients and rejuvenate your body with life-giving energy. No more zombie mornings and midafternoon energy slumps for you!

In addition to cutting out sugar, avoid caffeine and tobacco. Again, as you start giving your body the vital nutrients it requires from fresh Sipping Skinny juices and smoothies, you will find you no longer need those temporary and ultimately harmful pick-me-ups. Make sure you're consuming healthy fats like omega-3s, which have been shown to improve insulin sensitivity.[7]

Get adequate sleep. One study showed that even one night of partial sleep deprivation can promote insulin resistance.[8] If you are chronically sleep-deprived, you need to promptly address this problem.

Finally, get some exercise in at least three or four times per week. Exercising helps counteract insulin resistance because your body uses up glucose during physical activity without releasing additional insulin.[9] All of these lifestyle tweaks will help restore your cells' sensitivity to insulin and keep insulin production in check.

I would be remiss if I didn't also mention that reversing insulin resistance is key not just for weight loss and weight maintenance, but also for avoiding disease. Insulin resistance greatly increases the risk of developing type 2 diabetes and metabolic syndrome, and it remains a symptom of both conditions. Most people are familiar with type 2 diabetes and understand that it is defined by chronically high blood sugar levels and a dysfunctional production of and response to insulin. Perhaps less familiar, metabolic syndrome refers to a combination of symptoms that increase one's risk of not only diabetes but heart disease and stroke as well. Those symptoms include high blood sugar, body fat concentrated around the waist, high blood pressure, and abnormal cholesterol or triglyceride levels.[10]

Bottom line: Treat insulin resistance as a serious warning sign. Allow the Sipping Skinny program to help you reverse it before it develops into something more serious. If you already have type 2 diabetes or metabolic syndrome, Sipping Skinny can still help restore healthy blood sugar levels and reduce abdominal body fat, but understand it may just take a little longer. Make consistency your friend and Sip Skinny every day.

HAVE YOU BEEN DUPED BY
DIET SWEETENERS?

Many people think they're getting away with something when they drink diet sodas, use zero-calorie sweeteners in their coffee or tea, or eat sugar-free candy. After all, artificial sweeteners have long been marketed toward people who are concerned with their weight. But do they actually work?

A Purdue University study released in the February 2008 edition of the journal *Behavioral Neuroscience* found that rats gained more weight when they were fed diets with saccharin than rats that were fed diets containing sugar.[11]

In a 2012 study published in *PLOS ONE*, the results showed that over time male mice fed diets that included the artificial sweetener aspartame experienced elevated fasting blood glucose levels, a decrease in insulin sensitivity, and weight gain, including new deposits of deep tissue abdominal fat, called visceral fat.[12] Visceral fat is associated with insulin resistance, an increased risk for metabolic syndrome, and by extension, an increased risk for type 2 diabetes, heart disease, and stroke. Yikes!

The effects of saccharin and aspartame were examined together in a 2013 study published in *Appetite* magazine in which a control group of rats were given sugar for comparison. The conclusion? Adding either saccharin or aspartame to the rats' diet caused them to gain more weight than the rats being fed sugar.[13]

What about the all-too-popular Splenda? In 2008 the *Journal of Toxicology and Environmental Health* studied rats fed diets with Splenda and found that it significantly reduced the good bacteria in the intestines, created a more acidic environment in the intestines, and contributed to increases in body weight.[14]

In addition to these findings, many researchers have found evidence in their studies that suggest diet sweeteners change brain chemistry, alter metabolism, and negatively affect the body's microbiome. There is also the theory that consuming diet drinks and products causes people to gain weight by psychologically tricking them into consuming more food and/or higher-calorie food. It's become a comical stereotype to hear the guy next to you ordering a double cheeseburger, large fries, and (say it with me) a Diet Coke. Or the lady in front of you ordering a large sugar-free nonfat vanilla latté—with a pastry on the side. It is not uncommon for people to use their perceived good choices or behaviors as justification for committing bad ones, as if the good cancels out the bad. But more often than not, artificial sweeteners simply do not encourage healthy or even completely sugar-free eating. And they definitely don't contribute to a slimmer waist.

All things considered, it is best to avoid artificial sweeteners entirely, which includes aspartame (Equal, NutraSweet, NatraTaste Blue), sucralose (Splenda), saccharin (Sweet 'N Low, Sweet Twin, Necta Sweet), acesulfame potassium (Sunette, Equal Spoonful, Sweet One), and neotame. Artificial sweeteners are just that: artificial. Not natural. They are substances that have been engineered in laboratories by people in white coats. The body was not designed to take in foreign substances that have forcibly undergone molecular changes. To put it in no uncertain terms, artificial sweeteners mean toxicity! If you want to lose weight, but moreover if you want to be healthy, heed the studies that continue to uncover the damage that artificial sweeteners inflict, and don't put yourself at risk.

ALAS, COULD IT BE THY THYROID?

The thyroid releases hormones to regulate important body functions, including metabolism. If the thyroid doesn't produce enough hormones, a condition called hypothyroidism, you may experience some of the most common symptoms such as difficulty losing weight and weight gain. This is because people with underactive thyroids often have a very low basal metabolic rate, so even if they attempt to diet, their metabolisms slow down the more they restrict their calories. Hence, the dreaded weight loss plateau or—worse!—weight gain, even when cutting back. (Weight gain can also sometimes occur if the thyroid produces too many hormones, known as hyperthyroidism, but it's not as common.)

Sad but true, hypothyroidism and weight gain are seen more in women than men, and thyroid issues and weight gain often occur simultaneously with menopause. There are several reasons thyroid dysfunction rears its ugly head more often in women than men:

- Women are more prone to dieting than men. This is often of the "yo-yo" variety, vacillating between strict calorie reduction and just-as-extreme calorie binges once the feeling of constant restriction and deprivation grows old. This back-and-forth pattern slows down the metabolic rate and ultimately undermines the metabolism, especially during perimenopause.

- According to the American Psychological Association (APA), more women than men perceive their stress levels to be high.[15] Chronic stress overstimulates the adrenal glands to crank out more cortisol, which ends up exhausting the adrenals, compromising thyroid hormones, and causing fat to settle around the midsection.

- The APA also says more women than men (31 percent versus 21 percent) admit to eating as a way of coping with stress, including overeating or eating unhealthy foods.[16] This isn't surprising considering that the body seeks relief from stress and adrenal fatigue by craving refined sugar, carbohydrates, or starch to restore energy and increase feel-good hormones like serotonin. I know this one firsthand; when I face high-stress situations, I run for a potato, since sugar and refined flour foods are like poison for me. Female hormones like estrogen and progesterone were designed to exist in harmony together. Stress disrupts this delicate hormonal balance, which has a domino effect that upsets thyroid hormones and adrenal hormones.

Besides weight loss resistance and weight gain, other symptoms of a sluggish thyroid include fatigue, depression, cold hands and feet, a feeling of always being chilled, joint pain, muscle aches or cramps, brain fog, difficulty concentrating, forgetfulness, hair loss, brittle nails, dry skin, puffy face, constipation, frequent infections, hoarse voice, menstrual disorders, infertility, and low libido. If you identify with several of these symptoms and think a low thyroid might be your problem, you should ask to be tested by your doctor. If testing does not conclude that you have hypothyroidism, be aware that it is still possible your thyroid is not performing up to par, in which case you may find some of the recommended dietary and lifestyle changes below beneficial alongside a juicing or smoothie program like Sipping Skinny. (You can take the Thyroid Health Quiz on my website at https://www.juiceladycherie.com/Juice/do-you-have -thyroid-issues/. I also have extensive information on thyroid health in my book *The Juice Lady's Remedies for Thyroid Disorders*.)

Vicki Lost Six Pounds and Her Thyroid Is Doing Better

I have lost two pounds this week for a total of six pounds, an inch off my waist, and an inch and a half off my hips. I have a lot of energy. My thyroid is working better, and I am sleeping better as well. My pants are getting loose. I may be going down from a size four to a size two soon. I have noticed a difference in my skin too. It seems to be softer, and there also seems to be a reduction in the appearance of cellulite on the back of my thighs. I am planning to continue with the watercress smoothies and soups even after the diet is over to help keep my energy levels up.

OH, WHAT CAN YOU DO WITH A SLUGGISH THYROID?

If a low thyroid is dragging down your metabolism, you will want to focus on supporting your thyroid gland and increasing your overall health, starting with the following guidelines.

You need to get enough iodine, and I ain't lyin' to you.

Iodine is an essential element to thyroid hormone production. If you don't consume an adequate amount of iodine-rich foods, your thyroid may not produce enough hormones. Check your grocery list to see that foods like fish, seafood, sea vegetables, eggs, cranberries, spinach, and green bell peppers are regularly on it.

Also, say no to table salt and yes to sea salt. But wait, doesn't table salt contain iodine, and didn't I just say iodine is good for you? The real story about table salt (iodized sodium chloride, if we're being scientific) is that it's highly refined, bleached white, and devoid of naturally occurring minerals, including iodine. For this reason, isolated or synthetic iodine is added to table salt to replace the naturally occurring iodine lost during processing. This is not how salt or any other food was meant to be consumed. You will be much better off seasoning your food with sea salt, which contains naturally occurring minerals, including iodine. It is possible to get too much iodine, which can cause other kinds of thyroid problems, so consume salt moderately. Keep in mind that about half a teaspoon of sea salt gives you more than two-thirds the daily requirement of iodine for adults. If you struggle to get enough iodine from your diet, you can buy kelp tablets, preferably of the Icelandic or Norwegian variety since the waters there are purer. Or you may add a drop or two of liquid iodine each day to one of your Sipping Skinny drinks.

Minerals! Get your minerals here!

Besides iodine, there are plenty of other minerals and vitamins that encourage thyroid health, including zinc, selenium, manganese, chromium, B vitamins, vitamin C, vitamin E, and vitamin A. I recommend taking cod liver oil, which is a good source of vitamins A and D. You can even get it lemon- or orange-flavored for better taste. You may also want to look into a multivitamin or mineral supplement that contains selenium, which is necessary for the conversion of thyroid hormones, and chromium, which helps the body process carbohydrates, fats, and hormones.

A goitrogen named soy

Goitrogen isn't just a fun word to say, it's also a substance that interferes with the thyroid's absorption of iodine and hormone production. A big goitrogenic culprit is soy, which also contains hormone-disrupting phytoestrogens. These days soy derivatives are in a lot of packaged foods, even those marketed as health foods, so be sure to read ingredient labels before purchasing products. It has become standard for bottled salad dressings, sauces, and mayonnaise to list soybean oil as one of the first ingredients, and many products that boast of protein are made from soy. If you drink soy milk as an alternative to cow's milk, opt for almond, coconut, oat, hemp, or rice milk instead.

Fluoride is not your friend.

Like soy, fluoride also gets in the way of the thyroid's absorption of iodine. Sodium fluoride, a synthetic waste by-product, is added to public water supplies nationwide, so you will want to avoid drinking tap water unless you have a water purification system that removes fluoride. You will also want to purchase fluoride-free toothpaste and skip the fluoride treatment offered at the dentist's office. It is a halogen that will replace iodine (also a halogen) in the thyroid.

Oh, coconut oil! How do I love thee? Let me count the ways.

Virgin coconut oil is a heart-healthy and liver-friendly saturated fat. It does not oxidize and turn rancid easily and can be safely heated at medium temperatures. It can sit on your shelf for as long as two years without degrading. Because the liver likes to burn it, coconut oil is unique in its ability to support a healthy metabolism and weight. And listen up! It's heart healthy. It's no wonder this natural fat has been used for generations in tropical areas with superior health results.

Polyunsaturated oils, on the other hand, are bad for you. Very, very bad indeed.

Frying oils like soy, corn, safflower, and sunflower (any combination of which may be relabeled "vegetable oil") oxidize and turn rancid easily. This damages the liver and impairs the body's ability to convert the thyroid hormone T4 to T3, a necessary process in order to transform fat into usable energy. If T4 is not being converted to T3, excess fat doesn't get burned off and hypothyroid symptoms can develop. Bottom line: Avoid fried foods, fast food, packaged snack foods, store-bought baked goods, most store-bought salad dressings, and anything else that contains polyunsaturated oils or hydrogenated oils. Instead, cook and bake at home with coconut oil, along with extra-virgin olive oil and grapeseed oil. Your liver and thyroid will thank you for it, not to mention your waistline.

ARE YOU STUCK ON THE
STRESS EXPRESS?

I've already mentioned that stress activates the adrenal glands to release cortisol in the body. This triggers a surge of blood sugar, quickly followed by insulin, to put the body into fight-or-flight mode. Stress and cortisol are your friends if you need to quickly reach over to keep a child from grabbing something hot or if you need to run away from a mad dog that's chasing you. But there is no question that chronic stress is the enemy of weight loss. Chronic stress can come in many forms—from one's daily job, writing a book, taking care of an infant or elderly parent, having financial difficulties, or coping with the loss of a loved one. In any case, chronic stress exhausts the adrenals, compromises thyroid hormones, leads to insulin resistance, sparks cravings for processed sugar and carbohydrates, and activates fat storage, especially around the midsection. Basically, everything that you don't want when trying to lose weight.

Whereas stress promotes weight loss resistance and weight gain, relaxation does the opposite by putting your body in a state where it feels safe. Then it doesn't need to protect itself with blood sugar and insulin spikes and by storing away fat. If you're someone who feels guilty taking some time out for yourself, know that it is a matter of health and not selfishness or laziness. Active relaxation helps reduce inflammation, turns off your body's fat-storage mechanism, and helps maintain steady blood sugar levels. This is truly essential not just for weight loss but also for your psychological and emotional well-being. Take the time to care for your body and mind.

*Arlene Got Rid of the Depression and
Fatigue Caused by Stress*

Experiencing so much energy that I just can't seem to stop...

I am in my late thirties. While generally healthy, I have been battling depression/fatigue over the last nine months after a major setback [in career]. I've attributed the problem to mental/emotional shock and stress and sought improvement through exercise and spiritual discipline. It had not occurred to me that a HEALTHFUL DIET could be the key to completely reverse the gloom. I'm just truly thankful to Cherie and all of you ladies to be included in this awesome group!

TO SLEEP, PERCHANCE TO LOSE—AY, THERE'S THE RUB

We've all been told we should be getting seven to nine hours of sleep every night. Intellectually, we know that sleep is important. And yet for many of us, it's the first thing we sacrifice when we feel like we have too much work to do, or when we crave downtime at the end of the day to decompress from all the work we just did. But perhaps we would get more serious about prioritizing sleep if we truly understood the important role that it plays in weight control and weight loss.

Time and again, research has shown that partial sleep deprivation (typically defined as less than seven hours of sleep a night) leads to weight gain. But this goes beyond staying up past our bedtimes and giving in to a case of the "midnight munchies." That causes weight gain too, but we also have two critical hormones that come into play when it comes to controlling our appetites, and both are affected by sleep, or lack thereof.

Allow me to introduce you to leptin and ghrelin. Leptin suppresses appetite by making you feel satisfied, and ghrelin increases appetite by making you feel hungry. When we don't get adequate sleep, leptin levels decrease and ghrelin levels increase, which means that we feel compelled to eat more, even when we've already received a proper amount of food. What's more, when we have been deprived of sleep, we are more likely to crave simple carbohydrates and high-calorie foods.

One extensive study presented at the 2006 American Thoracic

Society International Conference revealed some rather startling insights into the relationship between partial sleep deprivation and weight gain. The Nurses' Health Study included just over 68,000 female participants, ages forty to sixty-five, who were asked to record, among other things, the duration of a typical night's sleep for them and their weight. The women recorded this information every two years over a sixteen-year period.

The study found that middle-aged women who sleep only five hours a night are 32 percent more likely to gain thirty-three pounds or more and 15 percent more likely to become obese than those who get seven hours of sleep a night.[17]

Here's the first interesting point to note: Women who sleep six hours a night are only 12 percent more likely to gain thirty-three pounds or more and only 6 percent more likely to become obese than those who sleep seven hours a night. Just by increasing the duration of sleep by one hour a night (from five hours to six hours), the likelihood of gaining significant weight drops by 20 percent and the likelihood of becoming obese falls by almost 10 percent.

The second interesting point to note is the fact that the women who slept less in this particular study did not eat more than their counterparts. In fact, they ate less. This suggests that leptin and ghrelin levels and their correlation to appetite don't always tell the whole story. The study's leader, Dr. Sanjay Patel, commented on the surprising data by suggesting that "sleeping deprivation may cause changes in a person's basal metabolic rate."[18] Cortisol production is also a likely factor, since we know lack of sleep inflicts stress on the body and raises cortisol levels, which leads to insulin resistance and weight gain.

If you've ever regarded sleep as an expendable activity in the context of your busy life, please think again—especially if the scale is not budging despite your best efforts. Sleep's effect on weight cannot be understated, as it influences blood sugar levels, insulin resistance, cortisol production, leptin and ghrelin production, food cravings, and metabolism as a whole. It may very well be the linchpin for which you've been searching.

But perhaps you want to get more sleep and can't. If that's the case, this next section is for you.

THE AMINO ACID PROGRAM: SLEEPING BEAUTY'S LITTLE-KNOWN SECRET

Ironically, while working on my sleep and weight loss book, I began having a terrible case of insomnia. A urinalysis test revealed that some of my primary brain neurotransmitters were severely unbalanced—specifically serotonin, dopamine, epinephrine, and norepinephrine. I learned that such an imbalance can require more than just diet to put everything back in order. Thankfully, I discovered that consuming amino acids specific to my needs works effectively and quickly. It only took about three weeks, and my deep, restful sleep was restored.

Neurotransmitters are natural chemicals that assist communication throughout the body and brain. The body manufactures neurotransmitters from the proteins we eat. Amino acids are the building blocks of protein, so it's not surprising that amino acids can help bring balance among the neurotransmitters that affect sleep. Serotonin and norepinephrine are two neurotransmitters that are essential for a quality sleep cycle. If serotonin and norepinephrine are not in balance, good quality sleep usually suffers.

You may be thinking, "Norepinephrine? Isn't that the creator of *When Harry Met Sally* and *Sleepless in Seattle*?" But you'd be wrong. That's Nora Ephron. Norepinephrine is one of our excitatory or stimulating neurotransmitters that should be high when we wake up in the morning and low by the time we're going to bed at night. Too much norepinephrine in the evening will cause insomnia—the hard-to-fall-asleep kind of insomnia. Or your adrenals may start pumping out cortisol and your body will kick in norepinephrine somewhere in the middle of the night or way too early

provides healing nourishment from nutrient-dense vegetables and fruit. You will be amazed by how much better you'll feel!

A DIGESTIVE DISORDER BY ANY OTHER NAME WOULD STILL SMELL AS…WELL, NOT VERY SWEET!

People who eat a whole foods diet and abstain from sugar, alcohol, and refined carbohydrates should lose excess weight and maintain a healthy weight quite naturally. If you've developed healthy eating habits but struggle with digestive issues and still can't seem to lose the weight, your body may not be completely breaking down your food and absorbing the nutrients. With poor digestion or a digestive disorder, you can be eating the healthiest food on the planet but your body still won't be able to receive all the nutrition it needs. This can cause nutrient deficiencies, fatigue, cravings, overeating, weight gain, and ultimately poor health.

Digestive disorders have many names but often share some of the same symptoms. The list includes dysbiosis (imbalance of bacterial flora); irritable bowel syndrome (IBS); gastritis; diverticular disease; intestinal permeability (commonly referred to as leaky gut syndrome), which leads to autoimmune conditions; and inflammatory bowel disease (IBD), like Crohn's disease or ulcerative colitis. Again, virtually all of these conditions are characterized by poor health and the greatest nemesis of weight loss: inflammation.

Perhaps you've never been diagnosed with a digestive disorder, so you don't think this section applies to you. But if you regularly suffer from such symptoms of poor digestion as gas, bloating, abdominal pain, acid reflux, constipation, diarrhea, or nausea, your digestive system is likely crying out for help. Whether or not you have a named digestive disorder, these symptoms suggest your organs of elimination need to detoxify. Otherwise, an impaired digestive system is a breeding ground for disease.

One of the best things a person with digestive issues can do is drink fresh vegetable and fruit juices, like those found in the Sipping

Skinny program. Juicing is especially effective for someone with impaired digestion because fresh vegetable and fruit juice doesn't need to be broken down by the digestive system as it is already in a liquid form the body can use immediately. We call this bio-availability. When you drink fresh vegetable and fruit juice, all the vitamins, minerals, and enzymes in the juice are quickly absorbed into your bloodstream and fed to your cells directly, providing the nourishment they most need. Sipping Skinny juices also alkalize the body, creating an environment that reduces inflammation, promotes healing, and improves immunity. You just can't go wrong with fresh juice!

If you want more specific information about detoxifying your intestinal tract, I recommend that you read my book *Juicing, Fasting, and Detoxing for Life*. In the meantime, besides juicing, you can improve your digestion by checking a few simple things off the list:

- Address food sensitivities. (Perhaps start with something like, "Greetings, Food Sensitivities!") Not surprisingly, many digestive disorders begin as food sensitivities, usually to grains, dairy, soy, and corn, the latter two being big GMO crops. Remove the offending food(s) and you will take the first step toward healing by reducing inflammation.

- Chew, chew, chew your food! It turns out Mom wasn't talking just to hear herself talk. Carbohydrate digestion begins after the first bite when amylase, the digestive enzyme in saliva, starts to work its magic. Chewing thoroughly mechanically breaks down food and increases the effectiveness of amylase and other digestive enzymes to continue breaking it down chemically. That's what I call teamwork!

- Drink plenty of water. If constipation is one of your issues, drink more water. It is critical to keep your bowels moving, or else waste will back up and breed unhealthy bacteria, causing inflammation in the intestinal lining. This can lead to intestinal permeability, also known as leaky gut syndrome. Also, the longer waste sits around in your gut, the more opportunities there are for toxins to recirculate through your body.

- Take your vitamins. Vitamin C and magnesium deficiencies can both lead to constipation. You can take vitamin C and magnesium citrate to improve bowel function.

- Fill up on fiber. Fiber is only available in food that comes from plants. It helps move out toxins, waste, fat, and cholesterol particles as it travels through the gut.[20] To get the most bang for your nutritional buck, try to eat five to nine servings of vegetables a day. Include all kinds of vegetables in a variety of colors, especially cruciferous veggies like broccoli, cauliflower, brussels sprouts, and cabbage—these all add a wonderful crunch to salads. You can also sprinkle ground flaxseed on your morning oatmeal to add a delightfully nutty taste, or blend in a smoothie.

- Feed your microbiota. Probiotics are strains of beneficial bacteria that promote a healthy intestinal environment. Look for probiotics that contain lactobacillus acidophilus and Bifidobacterium bifidum to keep bad intestinal bacteria in check. There are many other beneficial strains you can take as well.

- Take supplements to support digestive health. Digestive enzymes help your body to digest food when its own supply of enzymes is insufficient. You can also take enteric-coated peppermint oil to reduce abdominal pain, bloating, and gas.

CANDIDA ALBICANS: NOT ALWAYS A FUN-GI TO HAVE AROUND

Your intestines contain tens of trillions of bacteria that are designed to live in balanced, health-promoting harmony.[21] More often than not, Candida albicans is harmless yeast (or fungus) that exists as part of your gut microbiota. When a person is healthy, Candida albicans is not problematic because the good bacteria keep it in check. But if the population of "good guys" dwindles, then the gut can become overrun with yeasts and other bad bacteria, a condition known as candidiasis.

Candidiasis can begin quite simply with a diet high in refined sugar and carbohydrates, which yeasts feed on. Then if you add the use of antibiotics and other medications, including birth control pills, which kill off beneficial intestinal flora, you can quickly develop a Candida free-for-all in your gut.

According to the late Dr. Robert C. Atkins, about 20 percent of the people on the Atkins diet didn't lose weight because of candidiasis.[22] This was mainly because when yeasts proliferate, they generate intense cravings for refined sugar, refined carbohydrates, and alcohol. Essentially, they want to be fed, so they cause their host to desire their favorite foods.

Besides weight gain, candidiasis can cause food sensitivities, digestive disorders, poor immunity, yeast infections, ear and sinus infections, skin and nail fungal infections, fatigue, brain fog, depression, and joint pain. Some people even report feeling "sick all over." If you think you may have an issue with yeast overgrowth, I recommend you take the Candida Quiz in my book *The Coconut Diet*, or look for the quiz online.

SO YOU THINK YOU HAVE A YEAST PROBLEM

There are several things you can do to help reverse a yeast overgrowth and restore balance to your gut microbiome, but be prepared that symptoms may temporarily get worse as the yeasts die off. It's also possible to experience what is known as the Herxheimer reaction, which refers to adverse detoxifying reactions, like headaches or diarrhea, that result from the numerous yeast toxins, cell particles, and antigens that unhealthy microorganisms release as they are dying. They don't like to go down without a fight! But even if it gets worse before it gets better, remind yourself to trust the healing process. There is a light at the end of the tunnel, and that light is improved health and weight loss. You just have to take the first steps.

Go low-glycemic. (Try saying that ten times fast!) You will temporarily need to eliminate sugar of all types, grains, alcohol, fruit, other carbohydrates that quickly break down into sugar, even milk and dairy products—basically everything that Candida albicans is known to feed on. Lemons and limes are the only acceptable fruit for flavoring your juices and smoothies. Also, foods that contain mold or yeast need to be omitted, including dried fruit, peanuts, bread, cheese, and alcohol. We don't want to give the Candida more friends to play with.

Find ways to add virgin coconut oil to your diet. Among its many good qualities, coconut oil consists of medium chain fatty acids known to effectively kill Candida. A 2001 study at the University of Iceland found that "capric acid…causes the fastest and most effective killing of all three strains of C. albicans tested, leaving the cytoplasm disorganized and shrunken because of a disrupted or disintegrated plasma membrane. Lauric acid…was the most active at lower concentrations and after a longer incubation time."[23] Many other studies similarly affirm that the medium chain fatty acids in coconut oil work together to kill Candida, and without affecting beneficial bacteria.

Take digestive enzymes. Gastric hydrochloric acid, pancreatic enzymes, and bile all help keep yeast growth in check and prevent it from setting up shop in the walls of the small intestine. Insufficient digestive secretions can add to a yeast overgrowth problem. In order to treat chronic candidiasis, it is highly recommended that you supplement with hydrochloric acid (betaine HCL), pancreatic enzymes (proteases), and a lipotropic formula to improve bile flow (the formula should include choline, methionine and/or cysteine).

Give your immune system a boost. A dysfunctional immune system makes it easier for yeast to flourish, and overgrowth of Candida albicans further weakens the immune system. It's a frustrating cycle. If you are someone who comes down with everything that's going around, repeatedly suffering illness from viruses and chronic infections, your immune system is likely compromised and requires extra attention. Start by flooding your body with antioxidants. Take vitamin C to bowel tolerance, which means take enough to be effective but not so much that it gives you loose stools. If your stomach starts to gurgle, then you're approaching tolerance and your body has the amount of vitamin C it needs. Keep in mind, when the body is sick and immunity is low, the body will take a lot of vitamin C for healing. Don't be surprised if you end up taking thousands or even tens of thousands of milligrams of vitamin C in a day before approaching bowel tolerance. Take what your body needs.

Start popping probiotics. As you bump up your supply of good bacteria by taking probiotics, you will crowd out more of the yeast and bad bacteria. Depending on the severity of yeast overgrowth, it may be helpful to alternate between two or more probiotics to increase the variety of strains in your gut.

TWO OF A KIND
(NOT THE GOOD KIND):
CHRONIC FATIGUE SYNDROME
AND FIBROMYALGIA

Chronic fatigue syndrome (CFS) and fibromyalgia are disabling illnesses with many shared symptoms, including extreme exhaustion, muscle pain, sleep disturbances, and cognitive difficulties. CFS also involves hormonal imbalances like hypothyroidism, whereas fibromyalgia can cause stiffness and headaches. Weight gain often follows both conditions, a result of the hormonal imbalances, sleep difficulties, and reduction in activity levels due to fatigue.

Because the two conditions are so similar, the following remedies can help people suffering from either illness:

1. Give your adrenal glands some TLC. Together, stress and poor sleep deliver a one-two punch against the adrenals. The last thing you want to do is tax them further with caffeine, sugary foods, processed carbohydrates, and alcohol. Instead you want to nourish the adrenals and normalize blood sugar levels by consuming lots of vegetables (especially leafy greens), lean proteins, and healthy fats like avocado, extra-virgin olive oil, fish oil, and (what else?) virgin coconut oil. Be sure to get plenty of rest, listen to calming music, enjoy soothing essential oil aromatherapy, and take part in activities that relax you. You can also support your adrenals with supplements like vitamin C, vitamin B5, enzymes, pantothenic acid, rhodiola extract, schisandra, and holy basil.

2. Eat foods high in magnesium. Often people that suffer from CFS and fibromyalgia have low magnesium levels, which translates to low energy. Add some of the following foods to your grocery list and see if your energy doesn't perk up a little: leafy green vegetables like beet greens, spinach, Swiss chard, collard greens, and parsley, not to mention seeds, nuts, and legumes. (You can also take a supplement that combines magnesium and malic acid.)

3. Just a spoonful of virgin coconut oil…makes the fatigue go down. Taking a tablespoonful of coconut oil two to three times a day can add a little surge of energy in the body and help stimulate the metabolism. Additionally, if there are some microorganisms

wreaking havoc, like yeasts and viruses, the medium chain fatty acids in coconut oil will kill them off, relieving a little more of the immune system's load and freeing it up to function more efficiently. More than a few times I have been informed by fibromyalgia sufferers that going on the coconut diet took away their pain. (See my book *The Coconut Diet*.) What have you got to lose?

4. Detoxify your body. I know firsthand how important it is to cleanse your body of toxins when you're under the thumb of either of these conditions. I used to suffer from a severe case of chronic fatigue syndrome that included chronic pain. I healed my body completely through juicing, detoxing, and dietary changes. You can learn about my story and my more detailed programs for these conditions in my books *The Juice Lady's Guide to Juicing for Health* and *Juicing, Fasting, and Detoxing for Life*. If you suffer from CFS or fibromyalgia, it is important that you start a cleansing program as soon as possible. Health and vitality await you!

CHAPTER 7

SIPPING SKINNY MENU PLANS

T HE SIPPING SKINNY Menu Plans are designed to help you lose the weight you want with a healthy lifestyle that I hope will become a way of life once you reach your goal. To that end, I've incorporated a variety of juices, shakes, smoothies, and soups along with flavored waters to help you sip your way to success. I have chosen different recipes for each day of your menu plan; however, you don't have to change recipes each day. If you find one you like, you can stick with it. Or you can omit any recipe you don't like or substitute one ingredient for another to suit your needs.

If you want more recipes for an extensive weight loss program, get my book *The Juice Lady's Big Book of Juices and Green Smoothies*. It has around four hundred juice and smoothie recipes. If you want more soup recipes, get my book *Souping Is the New Juicing*. For the main low-carb meal, I did not include solid-food recipes in this book because it's all about recipes you can sip (or slurp!). For lots of main course recipe ideas, I highly recommend my book *The Juice Lady's Anti-Inflammation Diet*. In the menu plan I will refer to some of those recipes in hopes of giving you an idea of the types of foods you can eat.

For each breakfast, you may have a juice and/or a smoothie. (The recipes listed below can be found in chapter 8.) And if you need

Lunch

- Creamy Cauliflower Soup

Midafternoon break

- Ginger Strawberry Cucumber Water
- Small bowl of kale chips

Dinner

- Spring greens tossed with lemon juice and olive oil
- Roasted Wild Cod with Olive Vegetable Medley

DAY 3

Breakfast

- Ashwagandha or rooibos tea (with a squeeze of lemon, if desired)
- Spicy Cacao Smoothie

Midmorning snack

- Juice of choice, such as The Natural Diuretic (optional)
- Half dozen sun-dried or naturally processed green or black organic olives

Lunch

- Energizing Carrot Cumin Cold Soup

Midafternoon break

- Cranberry Green Tea Spritzer
- Two tablespoons pumpkin or sunflower seeds

Dinner

- Chicken Curry Salad

DAY 4

Breakfast

- Barberry or mint tea (with a squeeze of lemon, if desired)
- Rockin' Green Smoothie

Midmorning snack

- Icy Lemon Fennel
- Celery sticks with one teaspoon of almond butter

Lunch

- Thyroid Detox Soup (you can eat as much soup as you wish)

Midafternoon break

- Apple Cider Vinegar Fat Blaster
- Dehydrated Onion Rings

Dinner

- Smoked Salmon Collard Wrap with Honeyed Carrots

DAY 5

Breakfast

- Pu-erh or matcha tea (with a squeeze of lemon, if desired)
- Rockin' Green Smoothie

Midmorning snack

- Ginger Lemongrass Iced Tea
- Twelve raw almonds

Lunch

- Southwest Pureed Black Bean Soup (you may have as much soup as you wish)

Midafternoon break

- Ginger Mint Cucumber Water

Dinner

- Mediterranean Chicken and Olives with Wilted Spinach and Escarole Salad

DAY 6

Breakfast

- Hawthorn berry or horsetail tea (with a squeeze of lemon, if desired)
- Rockin' Green Smoothie

Midmorning snack

- Parsley Pep

Lunch

- Broccoli Spinach Soup

Midafternoon break

- Rosemary Oregano Water
- Six Brazil nuts (rich in selenium)

Dinner

- Drink one glass of water with one to two teaspoons of raw apple cider vinegar
- Black Bean Burger (no bun) with Baked Corinader Brown Rice and Shredded Carrot Slaw

DAY 7

Breakfast

- Hibiscus or juniper tea (with a squeeze of lemon, if desired)
- Slimming Strawberry Smoothie

Midmorning snack

- Celery Delight

Lunch

- Tomato Fennel Soup

Midafternoon break

- Lemon Pear Basil Water
- One Granny Smith or Pippin apple

Dinner

- Nut-Crusted Chicken with Whole Roasted Cauliflower and Scallion Cabbage Slaw

THYROID DETOX WEIGHT LOSS PLAN

As you improve your thyroid health, your weight loss should improve. Many people like April are diagnosed with either borderline hypothyroidism or get no diagnosis at all but still have a sluggish thyroid that keeps them from losing the weight they want to lose. A slow-functioning thyroid makes weight loss difficult.

April Improved Her Thyroid Function

On my Watercress Soup Diet, April lost seven pounds. She says, "My blood tests have always showed border-line hypothyroidism, but I never wanted to start the medications the doctors recommended. I believe the watercress is helping and has made a huge difference in my sustained energy, in exercise, and in my weight loss."

THYROID DETOX SOUP

This is a good soup to detox the thyroid. Parsley and cilantro attract heavy metals, so eating them can help you detox heavy metals. But make sure you purchase organic. You don't want more heavy metals in your body.

2 Tbsp. coconut oil or extra-virgin olive oil
1 large onion, chopped
2 cloves of garlic, minced
1 cup chopped broccoli
1 cup chopped parsnips
3 carrots, chopped
½ cup chopped cabbage
1 cup chopped cilantro
1 cup chopped watercress
½ cup chopped parsley
½ small jalapeño pepper, minced
2 zucchinis, chopped
Assortment of fresh herbs to taste
¼ cup almond butter, creamy or crunchy
8 cups organic vegetable or organic chicken broth

In a large soup pot add the oil, onions, and garlic and simmer for five minutes or until onions are soft. Add the remaining vegetables, the almond butter, and the broth. Bring to a simmer—do not boil. Cover and let simmer for two hours. If you like a creamier texture, you can blend all or part of it.

THYROID DETOX MENU PLAN

TOXINS THAT IMPACT THE THYROID

Studies have linked mercury exposure with elevated thyroid antibodies.[1] From mercury in dental fillings (silver amalgams), vaccines, fish, and industrial use, many people have been exposed to mercury. Aluminum will also affect the thyroid, and it is a part of most of our daily lives. It is so important to consume foods that help you detox your thyroid gland.

Breakfast

- Thyroid Detox Smoothie
- Ginger Tea (and a squeeze of lemon is nice), or start your day with hot water and lemon, a good thyroid detox drink
- You can add an egg if you need more protein

Midmorning snack

- Parsley Tea
- Green Juice Thyroid Helper (optional)

Lunch

Thyroid Detox Soup (you can eat as much soup as you like)

Midafternoon break

- Golden Milk

- Two tablespoons pumpkin or sunflower seeds, or twelve nuts (optional)

Dinner

- Eat no gluten, dairy, soy, or sweets (except for the stevia allowed in Golden Milk)

- Choose a low-carb dinner such as one of the following:
    Baked chicken, veggies, and salad
    Main course salad, such as grilled salmon over greens
    Stir-fry with veggies and protein

ACCOUNTABILITY: A KEY TO YOUR WILD SUCCESS

I want you to keep track of everything you eat, each and every day. The diet diary I put together for you follows. If you don't want to write in the book, make copies. Just make sure that you fill this out every day. This is your first step in accountability, which makes a huge difference in whether or not you will succeed. I assume you will continue the program for more than one week, unless you only have a couple of pounds to lose, so you'll definitely want to make copies in this case. Each day, at the end of the day, take a few minutes to write down what you ate. Or keep your diet diary with you all day and note as you go. Write down every little thing you plop into your mouth. You may be surprised at what you put in your mouth—things that you don't even think about, like something from your coworker's candy dish or snack bowl. Writing it down makes it unavoidable—no more ignoring what you're *really* eating. Too often we take a bite of something and forget about it, or we grab a few nuts or a snack item while on the go. It's all the little things that add up to a bunch of calories we didn't even think about or plan on eating. Your notations will really help you make the changes you need.

At the end of the day, do your assessment. Did you drink enough water? What about tea with thermogenic effects; did you try one? Did you include metabolism boosters somewhere in your day? Did you eat snacks? What food choices did you make for your main meal? How did you start your morning? If your day didn't go well and you didn't get the nourishment you needed, you were probably starved by noon. How much food did you eat in the evening? If you assess your actions objectively, you can make positive adjustments that will move you forward toward your goal.

Join a group to be accountable to others. I run many weight loss groups throughout the year, such as the Watercress Soup Diet Challenge. The people who do the best are those who join one of my groups and are active on the private Facebook page, interacting with others in the group and joining the weekly teleconference calls. When you are accountable to others, you will do much better. And when you are sharing your struggles with others, the group support is very helpful. Many people have said the group support made a big difference in their success.

TAKE AN ASSESSMENT

My husband is a biofeedback therapist. He is always telling me that with weight loss, people need feedback. He says you must weigh yourself. Anything else is a denial of reality. So no matter how your clothes fit, you need to know your weight and measurements. Before you begin your weight loss program, weigh yourself. You don't have to weigh yourself every day, but do it at least once a week. Keep in mind that your scale might head in the wrong direction occasionally because you are burning fat, which turns to water, and water weighs more than fat. So before the water gets eliminated, the scale might bump up slightly Make sure you consume plenty of natural diuretics. (See recipes in chapter 8.)

Now, write down your weight loss goal for each week. Also, write down your goals for exercise—set your goal to exercise at least three times a week. What type of workouts will you do?

Weight
Starting weight: _____

Weight, week 2: _____

Weight, week 3: _____

Measurements

Starting measurements

Bust: _____

Waist: _____

Hips: _____

Measurements, week 2

Bust: _____

Waist: _____

Hips: _____

Measurements, week 3

Bust: _____

Waist: _____

Hips: _____

Size
Starting size: _____

Size, week 2: _____

Size, week 3: _____

Set your goals
My weight loss goal, week 1: _____

My weight loss goal, week 2: _____

My weight loss goal, week 3: _____

My ideal weight (ultimate goal): _____

My ideal measurements

Bust: _____

Waist: _____

Hips: _____

My ideal size: _____

My exercise goals: _____

_____

_____

DAY 1

Vegetable juice, glass 1: _____

Vegetable juice, glass 2: _____

Water (minimum eight 8-ounce glasses per day): _____

Herbal tea: _____

Green tea: _____

Supplements: _____

Food List

Grain: _____

_____

Vegetables: _____

_____

Fruit: _____

_____

Meat/Fish/Poultry: _____

_____

Fat: _____

_____

Other: _____

_____

Diet Diary

Breakfast: _____

_____

Midmorning Break: _____

_____

Lunch: _____

_____

Midafternoon Snack: _____

_____

Dinner: _____

_____

DAY 2

Vegetable juice, glass 1: _____

Vegetable juice, glass 2: _____

Water (minimum eight 8-ounce glasses per day): _____

Herbal tea: _____

Green tea: _____

Supplements: _____

Food List

Grain: _____

_____

Vegetables: _____

_____

Fruit: _____

_____

Meat/Fish/Poultry: _____

_____

Fat: _____

_____

Other: _____

_____

Diet Diary

Breakfast: _____

_____

Midmorning Break: _____

_____

Lunch: _____

_____

Midafternoon Snack: _____

_____

Dinner: _____

_____

DAY 3

Vegetable juice, glass 1: _____

Vegetable juice, glass 2: _____

Water (minimum eight 8-ounce glasses per day): _____

Herbal tea: _____

Green tea: _____

Supplements: _____

Food List

Grain: _____

_____

Vegetables: _____

_____

Fruit: _____

_____

Meat/Fish/Poultry: _____

_____

Fat: _____

_____

Other: _____

_____

Diet Diary

Breakfast: _____

_____

Midmorning Break: _____

_____

Lunch: _____

_____

Midafternoon Snack: _____

_____

Dinner: _____

_____

DAY 4

Vegetable juice, glass 1: _____

Vegetable juice, glass 2: _____

Water (minimum eight 8-ounce glasses per day): _____

Herbal tea: _____

Green tea: _____

Supplements: _____

Food List

Grain: _____

_____

Vegetables: _____

_____

Fruit: _____

_____

Meat/Fish/Poultry: _____

_____

Fat: _____

_____

Other: _____

_____

Diet Diary

Breakfast: _____

_____

Midmorning Break: _____

_____

Lunch: _____

_____

Midafternoon Snack: _____

_____

Dinner: _____

_____

DAY 5

Vegetable juice, glass 1: _____

Vegetable juice, glass 2: _____

Water (minimum eight 8-ounce glasses per day): _____

Herbal tea: _____

Green tea: _____

Supplements: _____

Food List

Grain: _____

_____

Vegetables: _____

_____

Fruit: _____

_____

Meat/Fish/Poultry: _____

_____

Fat: _____

_____

Other: _____

_____

Diet Diary

Breakfast: _____

_____

Midmorning Break: _____

_____

Lunch: _____

_____

Midafternoon Snack: _____

_____

Dinner: _____

_____

DAY 6

Vegetable juice, glass 1: _____

Vegetable juice, glass 2: _____

Water (minimum eight 8-ounce glasses per day): _____

Herbal tea: _____

Green tea: _____

Supplements: _____

Food List

Grain: _____

_____

Vegetables: _____

_____

Fruit: _____

_____

Meat/Fish/Poultry: _____

_____

Fat: _____

_____

Other: _____

_____

Diet Diary

Breakfast: _____

_____

Midmorning Break: _____

_____

Lunch: _____

_____

Midafternoon Snack: _____

_____

Dinner: _____

_____

DAY 7

Vegetable juice, glass 1: _____

Vegetable juice, glass 2: _____

Water (minimum eight 8-ounce glasses per day): _____

Herbal tea: _____

Green tea: _____

Supplements: _____

Food List

Grain: _____

Vegetables: _____

Fruit: _____

Meat/Fish/Poultry: _____

Fat: _____

Other: _____

Diet Diary

Breakfast: _____

Midmorning Break: _____

Lunch: _____

Midafternoon Snack: _____

Dinner: _____

GO FORTH AND SUCCEED

There is a quote (attributed to various figures) that I read often: "To get something you never had, you have to do something you never did."[2] You know what they say about those people who keep doing the same thing over and over again and expect different results—that's insanity! One definition of *insanity* is extreme foolishness.

If you want a new body, it's important to see yourself in a new way—as the person you choose to become. Today is the day for new actions. If you want to be successful with your weight loss, decide now what you will do differently, namely, things that you haven't done before. Make the choice to be consistent each day as you work toward your goals.

I want you to close your eyes for a moment. Can you picture yourself at your ideal weight? Start a goal-minded collage board. Cut out a picture of a person who resembles the weight you want to achieve. Put it up in a place where you can see it often. This storyboard of goals does work. I did a storyboard of pictures years ago when I set my career goals. I still display it in my office. I had a picture of a writer on the page with a goal of writing many books. To date, I've written thirty-four books. At the time, I had only coauthored one book. I put a picture of television on there because I wanted to do something in my field on TV; my undergraduate degree is in speech communications. To date, I've been on hundreds of talk and news shows, have made appearances in five infomercials, and have appeared on QVC regularly for thirteen years with the George Foreman grills and the Juiceman and Juice Lady Juicers.

Before I began working with George Foreman and the grills, I put a picture of George on my board; he signed it for me when I first met him in Las Vegas, where he was fighting and introducing the grill for the first time at the Gourmet Product Show. Several months later I became George's nutritionist, appeared in three infomercials with him, and began representing the grills on QVC. So as you can see, setting pictures before your eyes can have a tremendous influence on your success.

METABOLISM BOOSTERS

CELERY DELIGHT

1 cucumber, peeled if not organic
3 ribs of celery with leaves
¼ small jicama
½ organic lemon with peel
1-inch chunk gingerroot

Cut produce to fit your juicer's feed tube. Juice ingredients and stir. Pour into a glass and enjoy. Serves 2.

DANDELION LIME ELIXIR

1 bunch dandelion greens
½-inch chunk gingerroot
1 lime, peeled if not organic
1 cup coconut water

Juice the dandelion greens, ginger, and lime; stir in coconut water, and serve immediately. Serves 1.

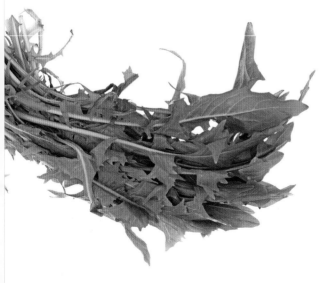

ENERGIZING WATERCRESS COCKTAIL

Watercress is one of the top plant sources of iodine, making it an excellent vegetable for the thyroid.

> 1 handful of watercress
> 1 dark green lettuce leaf
> 1 cucumber, peeled if not organic
> ½ fennel bulb and fronds
> 1 lemon, peeled if not organic
> ½-inch chunk gingerroot

Cut produce to fit your juicer's feed tube. Wrap watercress in lettuce leaf and push through juicer slowly. Juice all remaining ingredients. Pour into a glass, stir, and enjoy! Serves 1.

GINGER HELPER

> 1 cup carrot juice (5–7 carrots)
> 1 rib celery with leaves
> ½ green apple
> ½ lemon, peeled
> 1-inch chunk gingerroot

Juice all ingredients, stir, and enjoy! Serves 1.

GRAPEFRUIT FENNEL JICAMA COCKTAIL

1 red grapefruit, peeled
½ fennel bulb with fronds
2-inch-wide chunk of jicama, scrubbed

Juice all ingredients, stir, and enjoy! Serves 1–2.

LEMON BERRY LIMEADE

1 apple
½ lemon, peeled if not organic
½ lime, peeled if not organic
1 cup berries
½ cucumber

Juice all ingredients, stir, and enjoy! Serves 1.

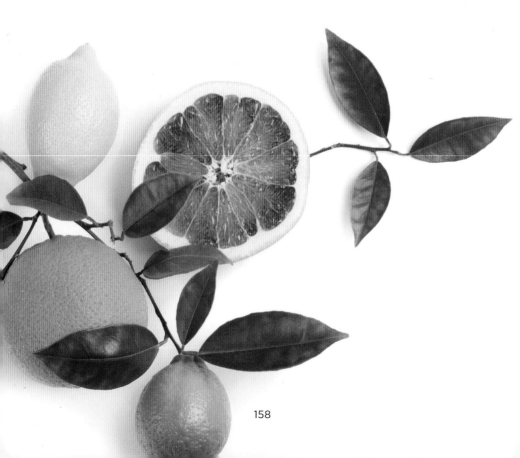

MINT SPINACH LEMONADE

1 small handful mint
1 handful spinach
2 apples
1 lemon, peeled if not organic

Cut produce to fit your juicer's feed tube. Juice all ingredients, stir, and enjoy. Serves 1.

MISTY MORNING

3 carrots, scrubbed well, tops removed, ends
     trimmed
½ red bell pepper with seeds and membrane
1 handful spinach
1 lemon, peeled if not organic

Cut produce to fit your juicer's feed tube. Juice all ingredients, stir, and enjoy. Serves 1.

RED CABBAGE COCKTAIL

3 carrots, scrubbed well, tops removed, ends
     trimmed
2 leaves red Swiss chard
½ apple
2-inch-thick wedge red cabbage
1 lime, peeled if not organic
1-inch chunk fresh turmeric (optional)

Cut produce to fit your juicer's feed tube. Juice all ingredients. Stir and pour into a glass. Drink as soon as possible. Serves 1.

WATERCRESS SKINNY SIPPER

1 apple
1 bunch watercress
2 ribs celery
½ medium cucumber
½ lemon, peeled if not organic

Cut produce to fit your juicer's feed tube. Juice all ingredients, stir, and enjoy. Serves 1.

DIURETIC COCKTAILS

ASPARAGUS LIMEADE

2 green apples
10 asparagus stems (use the tips for steaming)
1 lime, peeled

Cut produce to fit your juicer's feed tube. Juice all ingredients, stir, and enjoy. Serves 1.

CRANBERRY APPLE DELIGHT

2 apples (green are lower in sugar)
1 cup fresh cranberries or 1 Tbsp. unsweetened
    cranberry juice
½ cucumber, peeled if not organic
¼ lime, peeled if not organic

Cut produce to fit your juicer's feed tube. Juice all ingredients, stir, and enjoy. Serves 1.

CUCUMBER SIESTA

1 cucumber, peeled if not organic
1 handful cilantro
2 medium tomatoes
1 lime, peeled

Cut produce to fit your juicer's feed tube. Juice all ingredients, stir, and enjoy. Serves 1.

GARLIC LOVE

½ cucumber, peeled if not organic
1 handful watercress
3 carrots, scrubbed, tops removed
1–2 garlic cloves (no need to peel)
½ lemon, peeled
½ apple

Cut produce to fit your juicer's feed tube. Juice all ingredients, stir, and enjoy. Serves 1.

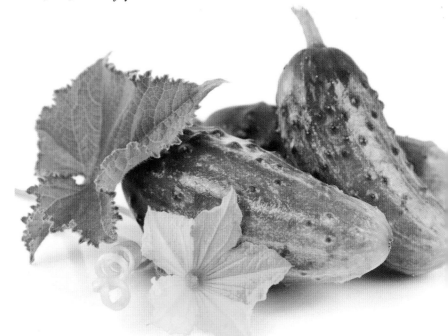

ICY LEMON FENNEL

1 fennel bulb with fronds
1 cucumber, peeled if not organic
1 lemon, peeled if not organic

Cut produce to fit your juicer's feed tube. Juice all ingredients, pour over ice, and serve. Serves 2.

PARSLEY PEP

1 handful parsley
½ fennel bulb with fronds
1 cucumber, peeled if not organic
1 lime, peeled

Cut produce to fit your juicer's feed tube. Juice all ingredients, pour over ice, and serve. Serves 1.

THE NATURAL DIURETIC

½ green apple
3 ribs celery
1 handful parsley
½ cucumber, peeled if not organic
½ lemon, peeled

Cut produce to fit your juicer's feed tube. Juice all ingredients and pour over ice. Serves 1.

TURMERIC TWISTER

1 cucumber, peeled if not organic
1 lemon, peeled
2 ribs celery
1 leaf chard
1-inch chunk fresh turmeric
1-inch chunk gingerroot

Cut produce to fit your juicer's feed tube. Juice all ingredients, stir, and enjoy. Serves 1.

WATERMELON CUCUMBER COOLER

1 strip of watermelon (about ⅛ of a small
    watermelon, or one long strip)*
1 cucumber

Juice ingredients and stir. Pour over ice. Enjoy. Serves 1–2.
    *To reduce the sugar content, juice the rind also. You can use a smaller piece if using the rind.

SLIMMING STRAWBERRY SMOOTHIE

> 1 cup unsweetened coconut or almond milk
> 1 cup frozen, unsweetened strawberries
> 2 Tbsp. flaxseeds

Combine all ingredients in a blender and process until smooth. Serves 1.

SKINNY SHAKE

> 1 cucumber, peeled and cut in chunks
> 1 rib celery, juiced or chopped into small pieces
> Juice of 1 lemon
> ½ teaspoon freshly grated organic lemon peel
> 1-inch chunk gingerroot

Place the cucumber chunks in a freezer bag and freeze them until solid. Combine the cucumber chunks in a blender with the celery, lemon juice, lemon peel, and gingerroot. Blend on high speed until smooth. Serves 1.

SPICE IT UP SMOOTHIE

> 1 cup fresh apple juice (1–2 apples)
> 4 oz. soft silken organic tofu
> ½ cup baby spinach, packed
> ½ tsp. cinnamon
> ⅛ tsp. black pepper
> ⅛ tsp. cardamom
> ¼ tsp. nutmeg
> Several drops liquid stevia

Add all ingredients to a blender and process until creamy. Serves 1.

SPICY CACAO SMOOTHIE

> 1½ cups unsweetened coconut milk or almond
>   milk
> ½ cup chopped kale
> ¼ jalapeño, chopped
> 1 tsp. ground cinnamon
> ¼ cup cacao powder
> Several stevia drops
> 4–6 ice cubes

Put all ingredients in a blender and process until well combined. Serves 1.

THYROID DETOX MOOTHIE

> 1 cup unsweetened coconut or almond milk
> 1 cup chopped spinach or watercress
> 1–2 cups fresh or frozen berries
> 1 tsp. pure vanilla extract
> 4–5 ice cubes

Put all ingredients in a blender and process until smooth. Serves 1.

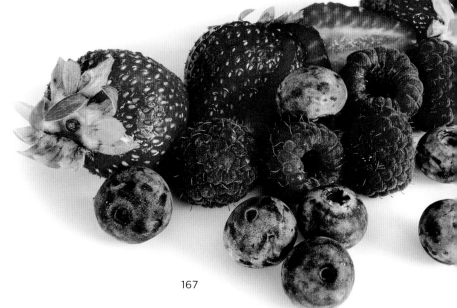

WATERCRESS BLUEBERRY SMOOTHIE

1 cup coconut milk (or other unsweetened plant
    milk)
1 cup chopped watercress
1–2 cups fresh or frozen blueberries
¼ cup chopped parsley
1 tsp. pure vanilla extract
6 ice cubes (optional, may not be needed if using
    frozen fruit)
Several drops of liquid stevia (optional)

Combine all ingredients in a blender and process well
until smooth and creamy/slushy. Serve as soon as possible.

WATERCRESS STRAWBERRY
APPLE GINGER SMOOTHIE

1 cup watercress
1 handful spinach
1 cup frozen strawberries

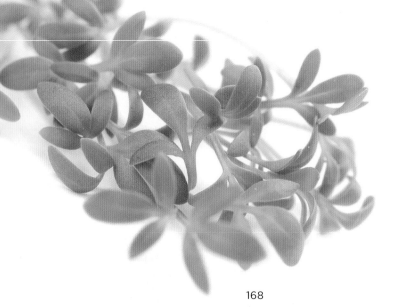

1-inch chunk gingerroot
½ cup fresh apple juice
½ cup plant milk (coconut or almond milk)

Combine all ingredients in a blender and process until smooth. Serves 1.

ICED LOW-CALORIE DRINKS

CRANBERRY GREEN TEA SPRITZER

2 cups water
4 green tea bags
½ cup unsweetened cranberry juice
3 cups sparkling water
Several drops liquid stevia

Heat water in a saucepan and add the tea bags. Let steep for 5 minutes. Remove bags and cool completely. Add cranberry juice and divide the tea into four different ice-filled glasses. Top with chilled sparkling water and serve. Serves 4.

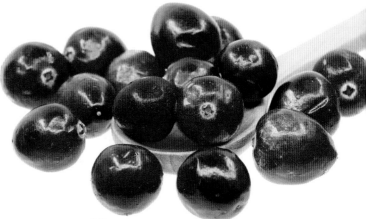

BASIC VEGETABLE BROTH

1 onion
2–3 carrots
3–4 ribs celery
4 sprigs fresh thyme
1 bay leaf
1 small bunch parsley
1 tsp. whole peppercorns
Sea salt to taste
Optional vegetable additions: fennel, tomatoes,
   mushrooms, parsnips

Roughly chop all the vegetables and herbs and throw them in a big pot. Cover them with enough water so that you can easily stir them. Simmer over medium heat and bring it to just under a boil. Once you start to see some bubbling at the edges of the pot, reduce the heat to medium-low. Cook for about an hour. Remove the pot from the stove and take out all the vegetables with a slotted spoon. Place your strainer over a big bowl and pour the stock through. Add the salt and pepper. Divide the stock into storage containers and cool completely. Freeze what you won't be using. Serves 6–8.

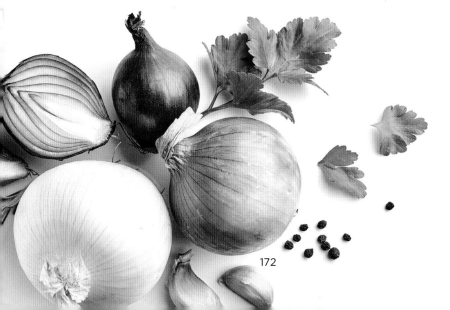

BONE BROTH
(FROM *SOUPING IS THE NEW JUICING*)

> 4–5 grass-fed beef bones, chicken bones, or any
>   mixture of bones from wild or pasture-raised,
>   healthy animals (if using beef bones, I prefer
>   meaty beef shank)
> Purified water
> 1 Tbsp. raw apple cider vinegar
> 1 carrot, chopped
> ¼ onion
> 1 clove garlic
> Sea salt and pepper

Place bones into a large soup pot or slow cooker. Fill your
pot with filtered water to cover the bones. Add the vinegar, carrot, onion, and garlic. Turn your heat on low for
the soup pot or set your slow cooker on low. Simmer for
24 hours. (I put my soup pot in the oven on 200 degrees
overnight.) Poultry bones can simmer as long as 24 hours,
and beef bones can simmer for up to 48 hours. Use tongs
to remove the bones, and then pour the broth through a
sieve into storage containers. Season with salt and pepper
to taste. Store in the refrigerator. It should keep for 5–7
days, or you can freeze it for later. Skim fat layer off the
top, if it forms. Serves 6.

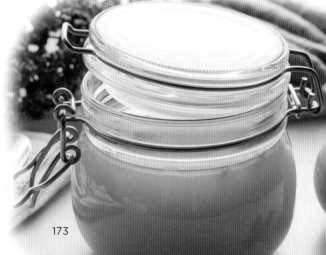

BROCCOLI SPINACH SOUP

2 Tbsp. coconut oil or extra-virgin olive oil
1 large onion, chopped
4 cloves garlic, chopped
½ tsp. sea salt, or to taste
Freshly ground black pepper, to taste
1 head of broccoli
6 cups organic vegetable or chicken broth
2 bunches spinach, trimmed
1 cup cilantro, chopped
½ tsp. finely grated organic lemon zest

Heat the oil in a large stockpot over medium-high. Add onion and chopped garlic and salt and pepper. Cook, stirring occasionally, until onion begins to soften, 3–5 minutes. Add broccoli and reduce heat to medium-low, cover pot, and cook, checking and stirring occasionally, until vegetables are very soft, 25–30 minutes. Add broth and increase heat to medium-high. Bring to a boil. Reduce heat and simmer, stirring occasionally, 10–15 minutes. Let cool slightly.

Blanch spinach and cilantro in a large pot of boiling salted water until bright green and just wilted, about 30 seconds. Drain and transfer to a bowl of cool water; let cool. Drain; squeeze out excess liquid. Either using an immersion blender or working in batches with a standard blender, purée soup base and blanched spinach and cilantro in a blender until very smooth and creamy. Pour soup back into pot and thin with broth as needed. Stir in the lemon zest and season with salt and pepper as desired. Serves 4.

CREAMY CAULIFLOWER SOUP

According to the *Journal of Nutrition*, blended soups may help diners feel full longer.

    2 Tbsp. extra-virgin olive oil or coconut oil
    2 tsp. minced garlic (2 cloves)
    2 cups onions, chopped
    1 tsp. sea salt, or to taste
    1 large head cauliflower, chopped
    7 cups vegetable or low sodium chicken broth
    ¼ cup raw cashews
    2 Tbsp. chopped green onions (optional)
    Grated nutmeg (optional)

Heat the oil in a large stockpot over medium heat and sauté the garlic, onions, and half the salt for about 3 minutes, or until the vegetables are soft. Add the cauliflower and sauté for another 3 minutes. Add the broth, increase the heat to high, and bring just to a boil. Reduce the heat to medium-low and simmer for 20 to 30 minutes, or until the cauliflower is completely tender.

Remove the pot from the heat and allow the soup to cool slightly; stir in the nuts.

Ladle the soup into your blender in batches and process on high for about 1 minute, or until smooth and creamy.

Return the soup to the pot and warm it over low heat. Stir in salt to taste.

Ladle the soup into bowls and garnish with either chopped green onions or grated nutmeg. Serves 6.

ENERGIZING CARROT CUMIN COLD SOUP

1 cup carrot juice (5–7 carrots)
1 small avocado
1 tsp. cumin

Put all ingredients in a blender and process until creamy.
Serves 1.

SOUTHWEST PUREED BLACK BEAN SOUP

2 Tbsp. extra-virgin olive oil or virgin coconut oil
1 medium onion, chopped
4 garlic cloves, minced
2 carrots, scrubbed and chopped
2 (15-ounce) cans black beans, drained and rinsed
6 cups organic chicken broth
1 tsp. dried oregano
1 tsp. ground coriander
2 tsp. ground cumin
Dash of cayenne pepper
½ to 1 tsp. sea salt
Freshly ground pepper to taste
2 Tbsp. fresh lime juice
¼ cup cilantro, chopped

In a large soup pan heat the oil over medium heat. Add the
onions and sauté for 3 minutes, or until soft. Add the garlic
and carrots and cook for about 8 minutes. Do not brown.

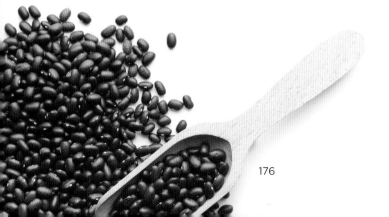

Add the black beans, chicken broth, oregano, coriander, cumin, cayenne pepper, and salt, and bring to a boil. Reduce the heat, cover, and simmer gently for about 15 minutes.

You can purée the soup using a handheld immersion blender, or ladle the soup in batches into a standard blender and process until smooth and creamy. Stir in the lime juice and season with salt and pepper to taste. Ladle the soup into bowls, garnish with cilantro and serve. Serves 4.

TOMATO FENNEL SOUP

2 Tbsp. coconut or extra-virgin olive oil
½ onion, chopped
1 bulb fennel, chopped
2 ribs celery, chopped
1 clove garlic, minced
1 (14.5-ounce) can diced tomatoes
2 cups organic vegetable or chicken broth
2 Tbsp. chopped fresh basil
2 Tbsp. chopped fresh parsley
½ tsp. sea salt, or to taste
Black pepper to taste

In a large stockpot, heat oil over medium-high heat. Add onion and sauté for 3 minutes, or until soft. Stir in fennel, celery, and garlic and sauté until tender, about 10 minutes. Pour tomatoes and broth over vegetable mixture and simmer for 5 minutes. Remove from heat and add basil and parsley. Cool soup slightly.

Ladle soup into a standard blender in batches or use an immersion blender. Puree until smooth. Season with salt and pepper to taste. Serves 4.

WATERCRESS WEIGHT LOSS SOUP

This soup can also be used for detox (adapted from Watercress Detox Soup in *Souping Is the New Juicing*).

2 Tbsp. coconut oil
2 cups sweet onion, diced
1 cup celery, diced
1 tsp. sea salt to taste
4 medium zucchini, diced (yields about 8 cups)
1 cup mushrooms, chopped
4 cups vegetable, chicken, or bone broth
¼–⅓ cup unsweetened almond butter, creamy or
    crunchy
2 cups watercress, chopped
2 tsp. fresh lemon juice (⅓ lemon, juiced)
Freshly ground pepper to taste

In a medium to large soup pot over medium heat, heat the oil and sauté the onion and celery with half the salt for about 5 minutes, or until translucent. Add the zucchini and mushrooms and sauté for 3 minutes. Add the broth and the other ½ teaspoon salt.

Stir in the almond butter until well combined. Increase the heat to high and bring to a boil. Reduce the heat to low and simmer for about 5 minutes or until the zucchini is tender. Add the watercress and let it simmer for about 5 minutes. Turn off the heat and cool the soup slightly. Stir in the lemon juice. Return the soup to the soup pot, season to taste, and warm over low heat. Serves 4.

Note: I have blended this soup on low so it's slightly chunky. I've also blended it on high so it's very creamy. I can't decide which I like more. You can add garlic, curry, or chopped scallions for variations.

WATERCRESS WRINKLE-FIGHTING SOUP

  1 Tbsp. extra-virgin olive oil or virgin coconut oil
  ½ cup chopped onions
  1–2 cloves garlic
  4 cups chicken broth or bone broth (vegetarians
      can use vegetable broth)
  1 medium head cauliflower, chopped (about
      1½ lbs.)
  2 cups watercress, chopped
  2 Tbsp. almond butter (crunchy or creamy)
  Sea salt and pepper to taste

Add oil to a stockpot and warm over low heat. Add the onions and garlic and sauté until soft (about 3 minutes). Add the broth and cauliflower and increase heat to medium-high. Bring to a boil, then cover and simmer over medium-low until vegetables are tender (about 20 minutes). Add the watercress until wilted, and stir in the almond butter; cook for about 1 minute and puree with an immersion blender or pour in batches into your blender and process until smooth. Season with salt and pepper to taste.

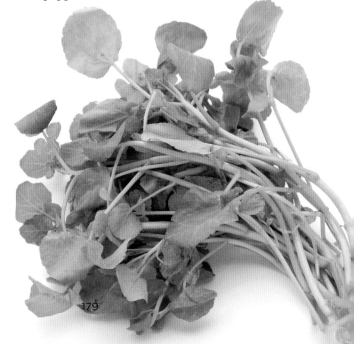

WEIGHT LOSS ELIXIRS
AND FLAVORED WATERS

APPLE CIDER VINEGAR FAT BLASTER

Make sure the apple cider vinegar is raw. Bragg's is the brand I use.

1 qt. purified water
2 Tbsp. apple cider vinegar
2 Tbsp. lemon juice
1 tsp. ground ginger
½ tsp. cinnamon
Dash of cayenne pepper
Several drops of stevia to taste

Mix all ingredients together. Drink a glass 20 minutes before a meal.

APPLE ROSEMARY WATER

½ apple, thinly sliced
2 sprigs rosemary
Pinch sea salt

Mix all ingredients in 2 quarts of purified water and chill.

BLUEBERRY LAVENDER WATER

½ cup blueberries
2 Tbsp. lavender flowers

Mix ingredients in 2 quarts of purified water and chill.

CUCUMBER MINT WATER

1 cucumber, thinly sliced, peeled if not organic
Several mint leaves
Pinch sea salt

Mix all ingredients in 2 quarts of purified water and chill.

FLAT BELLY CUCUMBER
STRAWBERRY BASIL WATER

½ cucumber, sliced, peeled if not organic
6 strawberries
2 Tbsp. basil

Mix ingredients in 2 quarts of purified water and chill.

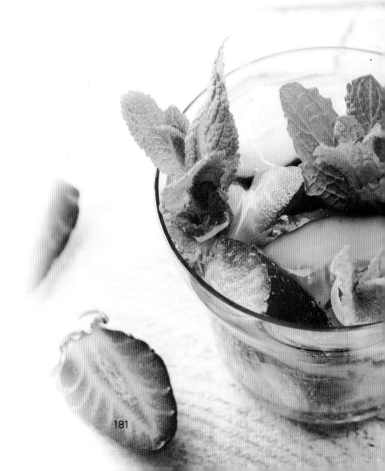

GINGER MINT CUCUMBER WATER

1 cucumber, thinly sliced, peeled if not organic
2 Tbsp. grated ginger
1 lemon, thinly sliced, peeled if not organic
1 lime, thinly sliced, peeled if not organic
Several mint leaves
Pinch of sea salt

Mix all ingredients in 2 quarts of purified water and chill.

GINGER STRAWBERRY CUCUMBER WATER

1 cucumber, thinly sliced, peeled if not organic
1 cup strawberries
2 Tbsp. grated ginger
Several mint leaves

Mix ingredients in 2 quarts of purified water and chill.

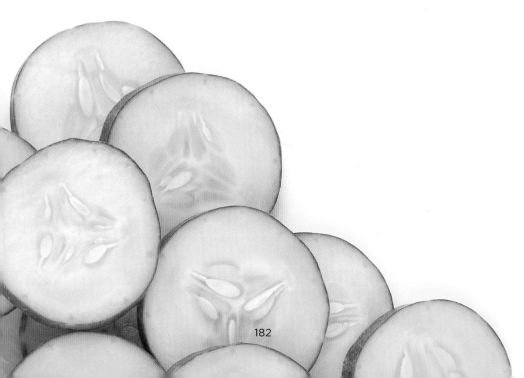

LEMON PEAR BASIL WATER

1 pear, thinly sliced
1 lemon, thinly sliced, peeled if not organic
Several sprigs basil

Mix all ingredients in 2 quarts of purified water and chill.

LIME LEMON PARSLEY WATER

Juice of 2 limes
1 lemon, sliced thinly, peeled if not organic
Several sprigs of fresh parsley

Mix ingredients in 2 quarts of purified water and chill.

ROSEMARY OREGANO WATER

2 sprigs fresh rosemary
2 sprigs fresh oregano
1 cucumber, thinly sliced, peeled if not organic

Mix all ingredients in 2 quarts of purified water and chill.

SKINNY DETOX CUCUMBER WATER

½ cucumber, sliced, peeled if not organic
½ lemon, sliced, peeled if not organic

Mix ingredients in 2 quarts of purified water and chill.

THYROID CLEANSE SIPPERS

GOLDEN MILK

This rich, detoxifying nut milk is made with turmeric and honey (or you can use coconut nectar or stevia). Turmeric helps fight inflammation throughout your body. If you have Hashimoto's, you have inflammation. And turmeric also helps detoxify heavy metals; there is often a heavy metal component with thyroid issues. In addition, turmeric helps regulate your metabolism and is very good for your digestion. Here's how to make Golden Milk.

First make a turmeric paste:

> ¼ cup turmeric powder
> ½ tsp. ground black pepper
> ½ cup purified water

In a small saucepan, mix ingredients well and then turn heat to medium-high and stir constantly until the mixture is a thick paste. This will only take a few minutes, so stir frequently.

Let the mixture cool and store it in a small jar in the fridge.

Next make golden milk:

> 1 cup of almond milk (hemp or coconut are also good options)
> 1 tsp. coconut oil or pastured butter
> ¼ to ½ tsp. turmeric paste
> Sweetener such as raw honey, coconut nectar, or liquid stevia to taste

In a saucepan, combine all the ingredients except the sweetener. Turn the heat to medium-low and stir constantly for 10 minutes. Don't allow to boil. Add the sweetener last, to taste, and remove from heat to cool for about 5 minutes.

GREEN JUICE THYROID HELPER

> 1 cucumber, peeled if not organic
> 2 ribs celery with leaves
> 2 leaves Swiss chard
> 1 cup watercress
> 1–2-inch chunk gingerroot
> Handful of parsley
> ½ lemon, peeled if not organic

Juice all ingredients, stir, and enjoy!

PARSLEY TEA

Parsley is an herb that binds heavy metals such as mercury and aluminum. Be sure to buy organic, because it binds these metals in nature while it's growing. It supports your pathways of elimination to keep your body clear of toxins. It is also a great anti-inflammatory herb. It is not good for pregnant women, however, as it is a uterine stimulant. Drink a cup of parsley tea midmorning.

Here's how to make your own parsley tea:

Start with about ¼ cup of fresh parsley in an infusion basket. Place the basket in a cup of hot water or a teapot with boiling water poured over it. Let it steep about 5 minutes. Remove the basket with the parsley. You may sweeten with a few drops of liquid stevia.

ADDITIONAL MENU PLAN RECIPES

BASIL STIR-FRY WITH CHICKEN

(from *The Juice Lady's Anti-Inflammation Diet*, page 122)

Fresh basil leaves make this recipe fresh and colorful. Use whole mint for a fun variation.

> 1 lb. boneless chicken (or tofu)
> 2 Tbsp. grape-seed oil or coconut oil
> 1-inch-piece minced ginger
> 2 cloves garlic, minced
> 2 cups carrots, sliced on the bias
> 1 head broccoli, cut into florets
> 1 head bok choy, sliced on the bias
> ½ cup whole basil leaves, packed (large stems removed)
> 4 Tbsp. stock (chicken) or water

Marinade

> 1–2 Tbsp. tamari (or coconut aminos)
> 1 Tbsp. arrowroot (or tapioca flour)
> 2 Tbsp. rice vinegar

Cut chicken into 2-inch pieces less than ½ inch wide. Mix the marinade in a bowl with a whisk to blend. Marinate the chicken for 10–20 minutes.

Heat the oil in a large skillet or a wok over very high heat. When the oil begins to ripple, stir in the meat, leaving marinade in the bowl for later use. When meat begins to brown, add the ginger and garlic for 15 seconds, then add the vegetables.

Quickly stir the vegetables and chicken until both are done, about 3–5 minutes only. Stir in the stock or water and remaining marinade. Simmer for 1–2 minutes more.

Optional add-ins: 1 tsp. sesame oil, 2 Tbsp. agave nectar, 2 Tbsp. rice vinegar, 1 Tbsp. hot chile oil, ¼ cup cashews.

Serves 4.

BLACK BEAN BURGER (NO BUN) WITH BAKED CORIANDER BROWN RICE AND SHREDDED CARROT SLAW

(from *The Juice Lady's Anti-Inflammation Diet*, page 132)

BLACK BEAN BURGER

Forgot to soak the beans? It's OK; you can eliminate this step by using fresh kombu, a seaweed used in traditional Japanese cooking. The kombu deactivates the enzyme inhibitor phytic acid, which causes us to feel bloated if we do not soak beans. Cut a 3-inch-piece of kombu. Cover the beans and kombu in water, bring to a boil for 5 minutes, then turn off the heat. Drain 2 hours later and proceed to cooking the beans with the kombu.

> 2 cups black beans, cooked (*reserve cooking liquid*)
> ¼ cup extra-virgin olive oil plus more for baking sheet
> ¾ cup gluten-free all-purpose flour
> 1 pinch of sea salt
> ¼ cup chickpea miso
> 2 Tbsp. coconut oil
> 1 cup yellow onions, finely chopped
> 2 cloves garlic, minced
> 2 tsp. ground cumin
> 1 tsp. ground turmeric
> 1 tsp. ground coriander
> 2 Tbsp. lime juice
> ¼ cup cilantro, finely chopped
> 1 tsp. sea salt

Do ahead: Cook the beans, covering them with 1–2 inches of water above bean level. Bring the beans to a boil, skimming off foam with a wooden spoon. Lower heat and simmer for 45 minutes to an hour and a half, until the beans are soft.

Preheat the oven to 350. Lightly grease one baking sheet with olive oil. In a medium bowl, mash the black beans until thick and pasty. Stir in olive oil, ¼ cup flour, a pinch of salt, and the miso. Set aside.

In a skillet, heat coconut oil on medium-high heat. Sauté onions for 5 minutes, stirring frequently. Add garlic and spices. Add lime juice, chopped cilantro, and salt; stir well. Remove from heat.

Add the seasoned and sautéed onions to the mashed beans, adding a few tablespoons of the bean water if needed to achieve a smoother consistency. Stir in remaining ¼–½ cup flour and mix with hands until combined and mixture sticks well together.

Divide the mixture into 6 to 8 burger-size patties. Line burgers on the greased baking sheet and bake for about 20 minutes, flipping once. Freeze extra. Serves 6–8.

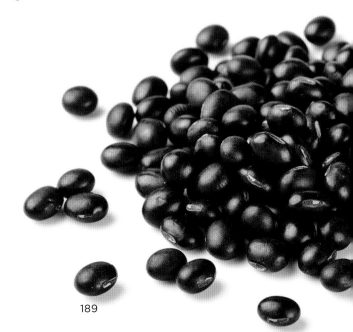

BAKED CORIANDER BROWN RICE

This is a great hands-off way to make aromatic rice using the oven rather than a pot or rice cooker. My favorite version includes a couple cinnamon sticks or coriander seeds! Baking the rice infuses the grain with a nutty aroma. If you soak the rice, reduce the water in this recipe to 4 cups and follow the shorter cooking time listed below.

> 6 cups water (4 cups for soaked rice)
> 2 cups brown basmati rice (or short-grain brown rice)
> 2 Tbsp. coriander seeds (or 1 cinnamon stick, or seasoning of choice)
> ¾ tsp. sea salt

Preheat oven to 375 degrees.

Bring the water to a boil in a pot on the stove. Use olive oil to oil a baking dish. Once water boils, add to baking dish, then stir in rice, seasonings, and salt. Cover with foil or a tight fitting lid (foil recommended)

Bake for 50 minutes (basmati rice) or 60–75 minutes for brown rice. If the rice was soaked, bake for 50–60 minutes.

Remove from oven to steam 3–5 minutes. Taste and serve! Serves 8.

SHREDDED CARROT SLAW

> 5 large carrots
> 1 large bulb fennel
> ½ head green cabbage
> ¼ cup lemon juice
> ¼ cup apple cider vinegar
> ⅓ cup extra-virgin olive oil
> Sea salt, to taste
> Freshly ground black pepper, to taste
> Optional add-ins: ¼ cup chopped parsley, 1 tsp.
>   ground cumin, 2 Tbsp. white sesame seeds, 1
>   Tbsp. raw honey.

Matchstick cut the carrots by hand or with a mandolin (little sticks). Finely chop the fronds of the fennel bulb. Thinly slice the fennel bulb and cabbage with a mandolin (or finely chop with a chef's knife). Toss all the vegetables together.

Whisk the dressing ingredients together, taste, and adjust. Toss dressing with the salad, and season to taste with salt and pepper.

Refrigerate for an hour before serving. Serves 4–6.

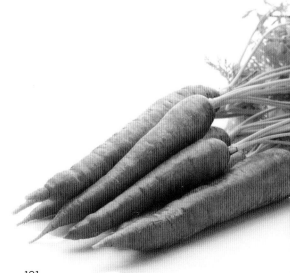

CHICKEN CURRY SALAD

(from *The Juice Lady's Anti-Inflammation Diet*, page 187)

½ cup Veganaise or mayonnaise
1 tsp. fresh lemon juice
2 Tbsp. curry powder
2 cups cooked chicken, chopped
¼ cup diced celery
½ cup chopped cilantro
¼ cup slivered almonds
1 head romaine lettuce or green leaf lettuce

Blend Veganaise or mayonnaise, lemon juice, and curry powder. Put the remaining ingredients (except lettuce) into a medium to large salad bowl and toss with the Veganaise or mayonnaise mixture. Chill at least one hour before serving.

Serve the chicken salad in the lettuce leaves or tear the lettuce and toss into the salad mixture.

Note: Walnuts may be substituted for almonds.

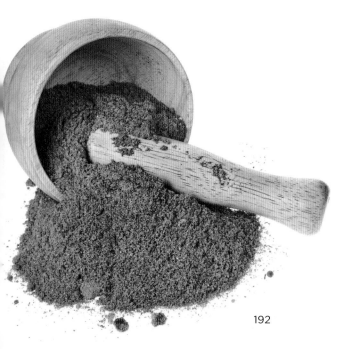

DEHYDRATED ONION RINGS

(from *The Juice Lady's Turbo Diet*, page 196)

> 3–5 onions (yellow, white, Walla Walla sweets)
> ¼ cup apple cider or coconut vinegar
> ¼ cup fresh lemon juice
> ¼ cup extra-virgin olive oil
> ½ tsp. Celtic sea salt
> Pinch of cayenne pepper
> 2 tsp. garlic, minced or pressed (optional)

Cut onions into thin slices and set aside. Add vinegar, lemon juice, olive oil, and sea salt to a blender and process until well combined. Then stir in the cayenne pepper and minced garlic, if using. Add the onion slices to the emulsion and marinate for several hours. Shake off excess marinade so that onion rings are not dripping with marinade. Place onion rings on dehydrator sheets for about 7–8 hours at 105 degrees or until crisp.

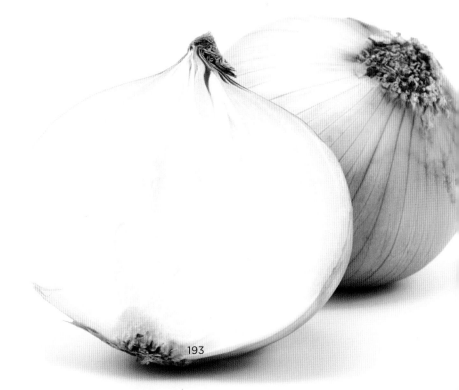

MEDITERRANEAN CHICKEN AND OLIVES WITH WILTED SPINACH AND ESCAROLE SALAD

(from *The Juice Lady's Anti-Inflammation Diet*, page 176)

MEDITERRANEAN CHICKEN AND OLIVES

¼ cup grape-seed oil
1 small yellow onion, chopped
5 garlic cloves, minced
1¼ lb. boneless, skinless chicken breasts, sliced
    into 1-inch pieces
1 Tbsp. fresh oregano, destemmed
⅓ cup pitted kalamata olives, coarsely chopped
1 jar artichokes in water, coarsely chopped
2 cups vegetable or chicken stock
2 Tbsp. red wine or red wine vinegar
½ tsp. sea salt
Freshly ground black pepper, to taste
¼ cup fresh basil, destemmed and coarsely
    chopped

Preheat the oven to 375.

Heat a heavy skillet that can transfer to the oven over medium-high heat. Add the oil, onion, and garlic with a pinch of salt. Cook for 2–3 minutes then add the chicken and cook until it begins to brown, about 4 minutes.

Add the remaining ingredients apart from the fresh basil, stirring to coat the chicken evenly. Cover and transfer to the oven to cook for 20–25 minutes.

Remove from oven and stir in chopped basil. Season to taste. Serves 4–6.

WILTED SPINACH AND ESCAROLE SALAD

> 2 Tbsp. extra-virgin olive oil
> ½ lb. spinach
> 1 head Italian escarole, chopped
> 1 Tbsp. raw honey
> ¼ cup dried currants
> ¼ tsp. sea salt

Heat a medium skillet over medium-low heat, then add the olive oil. Add the spinach and escarole in 2 batches; as the first batch wilts add the second in, when there is room.

When all the greens are bright and lightly wilted, add in the honey, currants, and salt. Sauté for 3–4 minutes, and season to taste. Serve the chicken over top of the wilted salad. Serves 4.

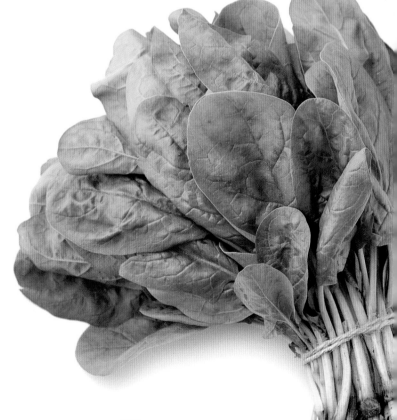

NUT-CRUSTED CHICKEN WITH WHOLE ROASTED CAULIFLOWER AND SCALLION CABBAGE SLAW

(from *The Juice Lady's Anti-Inflammation Diet*, page 81)

NUT-CRUSTED CHICKEN

This recipe satisfies the desire for crispy, crunchy, fried food without all the bad oils and white flour. I live in Oregon, so hazelnuts (filberts) are a favorite nut choice for me. Pecans and almonds are also fabulous in this recipe.

> 2 cups nuts of choice, finely ground
> 1 tsp. sea salt
> ¼ tsp. freshly ground black pepper
> 2 tsp. herbs/spices of choice (onion powder, garlic powder, paprika, oregano, etc.)
> 4 free-range chicken breasts, boneless, skinless, cut in tender-size strips
> 2 large eggs, beaten

Pour cup of nut meal into a bowl. Add salt, pepper, and enough seasonings until it tastes good to you. Dip the chicken pieces into beaten eggs. Next, lightly coat in nut/seasoning mixture.

Broil on high for 7 minutes, then flip and broil for another 5 minutes, or until juices run clear and there is no pink in the center. Serves 4.

WHOLE ROASTED CAULIFLOWER

2 whole heads of cauliflower, cut in half
¼ cup grape-seed oil
½ tsp. sea salt

Preheat the oven to 350 degrees.

Place the cauliflower halves on a lightly oiled baking sheet. Rub the remaining oil on the cauliflower and sprinkle with sea salt.

Roast in the oven for 1 hour. Serve warm or chill and toss in a salad. Serves 4.

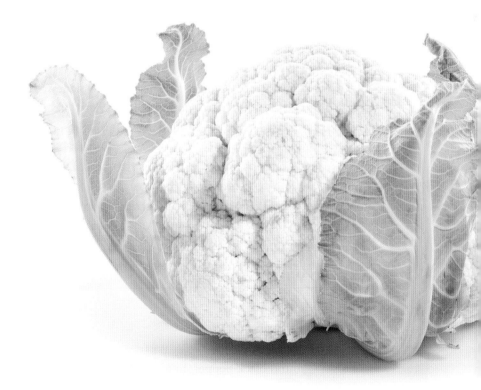

SMOKED SALMON COLLARD WRAP WITH HONEYED CARROTS

(from *The Juice Lady's Anti-Inflammation Diet*, page 84)

SMOKED SALMON COLLARD WRAP

1 large bunch collard greens (8 leaves)
1 avocado, mashed
3 Tbsp. lemon juice, to taste
½ lb. smoked salmon, flaked into pieces
1 cup sprouts
1 cup cucumber, sliced thinly
½ cup tarragon or parsley, chopped
Sea salt, to taste
Freshly ground black pepper, to taste

Assemble the wrap as follows: Destem collard leaf to remove hard central stem so that each collard leaf yields 2 collard wrap pieces.

Lay out the collard leaf pieces in a row and add mashed avocado and a sprinkle of lemon to each piece. Add smoked salmon, dividing equally over the avocado.

Add sprouts, cucumber, and tarragon or parsley over the salmon. Roll each piece away from you, carefully placing wrap seam side down, and repeat. Secure with a toothpick until ready to serve. Serves 4.

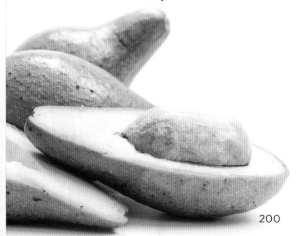

HONEYED CARROTS

1½ lb. carrots, rolling stew cut
½ tsp. sea salt
¼ tsp. freshly ground pepper
½ cup raw honey
2 Tbsp. coconut oil

Wash the carrots, then cut: slice on the bias, then roll the carrot away from you, then cut on the bias again. This should form a stew cut carrot. Repeat with remaining carrots.

Place carrots in a skillet and add water to cover halfway up the side of the pan. Cover and steam on high until most of the water evaporates and carrots are nearly steamed through, about 5–7 minutes.

Add remaining ingredients and lower heat to medium low, simmering for 5–10 minutes more until carrots are nicely glazed. Serves 4.

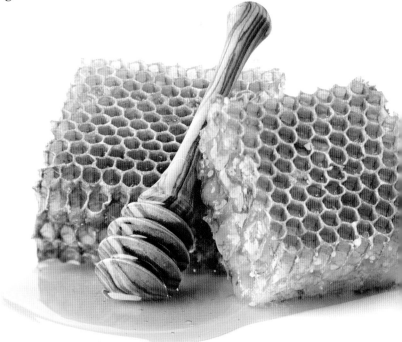

RESOURCES

Join Cherie's Juicy Tips Newsletter. Get a free recipe and 10 percent off your first order for signing up, and get recipes and healthy tips twice a week from America's Most Trusted Nutritionist. Go to https://www.juiceladyinfo.com.

Sign up now for your five-day guided juice fast, "The Juice Lady's 5-Day Juice FASSST," at https://www.juiceladycherie.com/Juice/fassst/.

Register here for Cherie's 30-Day Detox Challenge: https://www.juiceladycherie.com/Juice/30-day-detox/.

Don't miss the Watercress Soup Diet; go to https://www.juiceladycherie.com/Juice/watercress-soup-diet/.

CONNECT WITH CHERIE

Cherie's Websites

Visit https://www.juiceladyinfo.com, https://www.juiceladycherie.com, or https://www.cheriecalbom.com for information on juicing and weight loss.

The Juice Lady's Health and Wellness Juice & Raw Foods Cleanse Retreats

I invite you to join us for a week that can change your life! Our retreats offer gourmet organic raw foods, with a midweek, three-day juice fast. We present interesting, informative classes in a beautiful, peaceful setting where you can experience healing and restoration of body and soul. For more information and dates for the retreats, visit https://www.juiceladycherie.com/Juice/juice-raw-food-retreat/ or call 866-843-8935.

The Watercress Soup Diet

This three-week e-course, with a lesson each week, helps you lose weight with the Watercress Berry Smoothie, the Watercress Soup, and a low-carb main meal. You will get recipes, guidelines, and information about the program. You'll also get private Facebook coaching, group interaction, and a teleconference call each week with Cherie.

For more information, go to https://www.juiceladycherie.com/ or call 866-843-8935.

The Juice Lady's 30-Day Detox Challenge

This is a four-week e-course designed to help you rid your body of toxins, contaminants, waste, and heavy metals that can accumulate in joints, organs, tissues, cells, the lymphatic system, and the bloodstream. It can energize your entire body. You'll get an e-lesson each week, private Facebook coaching with Cherie, and a teleconference call each week where you can ask questions. For more information, go to https://www.juiceladycherie.com/Juice/30-day-detox/ or call 866-843-8935.

The Juice Lady's 28-Day Juicing for Weight Loss

This four-week course has eight downloadable lessons to help you lose the weight you want. For more information go to https://www .juiceladycherie.com or call 866-843-8935.

Nutrition Counseling

To schedule a nutrition consultation with the Juice Lady's team, visit https://www.juiceladycherie.com/Juice/nutritional-counseling/ or call 866-843-8935.

Scheduling Cherie Calbom to Speak

To schedule Cherie Calbom to speak to your organization, call 866-843-8935.

BOOKS BY CHERIE AND JOHN CALBOM

These books can be ordered at any of the websites above or by calling 866-843-8935.

- Cherie Calbom, *The Juice Lady's Guide to Fasting* (Siloam Press)

- Cherie Calbom, *The Juice Lady's Remedies for Diabetes* (Siloam Press)

- Cherie Calbom, *The Juice Lady's Sugar Knockout* (Siloam Press)

- Cherie Calbom, Abby Fammartino, *The Juice Lady's Anti-Inflammation Diet* (Siloam Press)

- Cherie Calbom, *The Juice Lady's Big Book of Juices and Green Smoothies* (Siloam Press)

- Cherie Calbom, *The Juice Lady's Remedies for Asthma and Allergies* (Siloam Press)

- Cherie Calbom, *The Juice Lady's Remedies for Stress and Adrenal Fatigue* (Siloam Press)

- Cherie Calbom, *The Juice Lady's Weekend Weight-Loss Diet* (Siloam Press)

- Cherie Calbom, *The Juice Lady's Living Foods Revolution* (Siloam Press)

- Cherie Calbom, *The Juice Lady's Turbo Diet* (Siloam Press)

- Cherie Calbom, *The Juice Lady's Guide to Juicing for Health* (Avery)

NOTES

CHAPTER 1 | SIP IT OFF!

1.   Josh Axe, "Which Protein Is Better, Whey or Soy?," DrAxe.com, accessed August 7, 2017, https://draxe.com/which -protein-is-better-whey-or-soy/.

2.   Jamie Oliver, AZQuotes.com, Wind and Fly LTD, 2017, accessed September 22, 2017, http://www.azquotes.com/quote /872840.

3.   As quoted in Richard Smith, "Let Food Be Thy Medicine…" *British Medical Journal* 328, no. 7433 (January 24, 2004): 0, https:// www.ncbi.nlm.nih.gov/pmc/articles/PMC318470/.

CHAPTER 2 | THE SKINNIEST LITTLE DRINK OF THEM ALL!

1.   Salynn Boyles, "Drinking Water May Speed Weight Loss," WebMD, January 5, 2004, https://www.webmd.com/diet/news /20040105/drinking-water-may-speed-weight-loss.

2.   Boyles, "Drinking Water May Speed Weight Loss."

3.   Boyles, "Drinking Water May Speed Weight Loss."

4.   "Frequently Asked Questions," Brigham Health: Brigham and Women's Hospital, accessed May 26, 2017, http://www .brighamandwomens.org/Patients_Visitors/pcs/nutrition/services /healtheweightforwomen/faq.aspx#protein.

5.   Fereydoon Batmanghelidj, "Hydration Is Vital for Optimum Health," accessed May 16, 2017, http://www.structural bodyworks.com/hydrateforlife.htm; see also F. Batmanghelidj, *Your Body's Many Cries for Water* (Falls Church, VA: Global Health Solutions, Inc., 2008).

6.   *CNN Health+*, "Expert Q&A: Can Drinking Lots of Water Help You Lose Weight?," accessed May 16, 2017, http://www.cnn .com/2009/HEALTH/expert.q.a/04/10/water.losing.weight.jam polis/.

7.   Janet Morrow, "Does Water Consumption Help You Lose Weight?" Hive Health Media, August 30, 2010, https://www.hive healthmedia.com/water-consumption-lose-weight/.

8.   Ingrid Macher, "Discover How Keeping Hydrated Can Improve Your Metabolism," Get Healthy, Get Hot, accessed May 16, 2017, http://gethealthygethot.com/2031/discover-how-keeping -hydrated-can-improve-your-metabolism/.

9.   From "Types of Covalent Bonds: Polar and Nonpolar," Exploring Our Fluid Earth: Teaching Science as Inquiry, accessed November 12, 2017, https://manoa.hawaii.edu/exploringourfluid earth/chemical/properties-water/types-covalent-bonds-polar-and -nonpolar; see also "Fact Sheet: DNA-RNA-Protein," microBEnet, accessed June 10, 2016, http://microbe.net/simple-guides/fact -sheet-dna-rna-protein/.

10. Joseph Mercola, "Villages in India Show the U.S. Just How Dangerous Fluoride in Our Water Is…," Mercola.com, July 20, 2010, https://articles.mercola.com/sites/articles/archive/2010/07/20 /indian-children-blinded-crippled-by-fluoride-in-water.aspx.

11. Joseph Mercola, "Bottled Water Poisons Your Body One Swallow at a Time," Mercola.com, January 15, 2011, https://

articles.mercola.com/sites/articles/archive/2011/01/15/dangers-of
-drinking-water-from-a-plastic-bottle.aspx.

12. Roy Speiser, "Why Toxins in Tap Water Are Damaging
Our Health," Honey Colony, March 1, 2016, https://www.honey
colony.com/article/toxins_in_tap_water/; see also Jeff Donn,
Martha Mendoza, and Justin Pritchard, "PHARMAWATER 1:
Pharmaceuticals Found in Drinking Water, Affecting Wildlife and
Maybe Humans," Associated Press, March 10, 2008, http://hosted
.ap.org/specials/interactives/pharmawater_site/day1_01.html.

13. Speiser, "Why Toxins in Tap Water Are Damaging Our
Health."

14. Melissa C. Navia, "Toxins in Your Tap," Detox My Water,
October 9, 2011, http://www.detoxmywater.com/water-world
/toxins-in-your-tap?page=0.

15. Navia, "Toxins in Your Tap."

16. Wendy Parrish, "Sun-Charged Water: Sun Power," Natural
FeetZonology.com, accessed June 11, 2016, http://www.natural
feetfootzonology.com/suns-power.html.

CHAPTER 3 | GAME CHANGERS: METABOLISM BOOSTERS AND WEIGHT LOSS HELPERS

1. Stuart Quan, "Too Little Sleep and Too Much Weight: A
Dangerous Duo," Harvard Health Publishing, October 7, 2015,
https://www.health.harvard.edu/blog/too-little-sleep-and-too
-much-weight-a-dangerous-duo-201510078396.

2. "The 55 Best Ways to Boost Your Metabolism," *Eat This,
Not That!*, accessed June 10, 2017, http://www.eatthis.com/best
-ways-to-speed-up-your-metabolism/.

3. "The 55 Best Ways to Boost Your Metabolism," *Eat This, Not That!*

4. Alexandra Sifferlin, "This Kind of Vegetable Can Help You Lose Weight," *Time Health*, September 22, 2015, http://time.com/4044476/veggies-fruit-weight-loss/; see also Monica L. Bertoia et al., "Changes in Intake of Fruits and Vegetables and Weight Change in United States Men and Women Followed for Up to 24 Years: Analysis from Three Prospective Cohort Studies," PLOS Medicine 12, no. 9 (2015): e1001878, https://doi.org/10.1371/journal.pmed.1001878

5. M. C. Kumar et al., "Acute Toxicity and Diuretic Studies of the Roots of Asparagus Racemosus Willd in Rats," *West Indian Medical Journal* 59, no. 1 (January 2010): 3–6, accessed July 4, 2017, https://www.ncbi.nlm.nih.gov/pubmed/20931905.

6. Salma Khan, "Revealed: the 5 Foods Which Naturally Enhance Weight Loss," *Daily Mail*, July 11, 2016, http://www.dailymail.co.uk/health/article-3684301/5-foods-naturally-enhance-weight-loss-snack-dark-chocolate-munch-celery-sticks-eat-salmon.html.

7. "Lose Over a Stone in Six Weeks with the Watercress Soup Diet," Watercress Alliance, accessed June 9, 2017, http://www.watercress.co.uk/diet/watercress-diet/.

8. Cynthia Sass, "Eat This Green Veggie for Better Workout Results," *Shape*, accessed June 8, 2017, http://www.shape.com/blogs/weight-loss-coach/eat-green-veggie-better-workout-results.

9. Shivapriya Manchali, Kotamballi N. Chidambara Murthy, and Bhimanagouda S. Patil, "Crucial Facts about Health Benefits of Popular Cruciferous Vegetables," *Journal of Functional Foods* 4,

no. 1 (January 2012): 94–106, https://doi.org/10.1016/j.jff
.2011.08.004.

10. Bianca London, "Eat Your Way to a Facelift: Watercress Is the Latest Wonder Food in Battle Against Ageing," *Daily Mail*, October 12, 2012, http://www.dailymail.co.uk/femail/article -2216852/Eat-way-facelift-Watercress-latest-wonder-food-battle -anti-ageing.html.

11. Mara Ventura, Miguel Melo, and Francisco Carrilho, "Selenium and Thyroid Disease: From Pathophysiology to Treatment," *International Journal of Endochrinology* 2017, https://doi.org /10.1155/2017/1297658.

12. "Studies and Research on Wheatgrass," Dynamic Greens, accessed June 12, 2017, https://www.dynamicgreens.com/en-us /studies-and-research-on-wheatgrass/page/4/; see also A. Schluter et al., "The Chlorophyll-Derived Metabolite Phytanic Acid Induces White Adipocyte Differentiation," *International Journal of Obesity and Related Metabolic Disorders* 26, no. 9 (September 2002): 1277–80, https://doi.org/10.1038/sj.ijo.0802068.

13. Victor L. Fulgoni III, Mark Dreher, and Adrienne J. Davenport, "Avocado Consumption Is Associated with Better Diet Quality and Nutrient Intake, and Lower Metabolic Syndrome Risk in US Adults: Results from the National Health and Nutrition Examination Survey (NHANES) 2001–2008," *Nutrition Journal* 12 (2013): 1, https://doi.org/10.1186/1475-2891-12-1.

14. Helen Nichols, "30 Foods That Can Help Lose Weight (Science-Backed)," Well-Being Secrets, accessed June 12, 2017, http://www.well-beingsecrets.com/weight-loss-foods/; see also Michelle Wien et al., "A Randomized 3x3 Crossover Study to Evaluate the Effect of Hass Avocado Intake on Post-Ingestive Satiety, Glucose and Insulin Levels, and Subsequent Energy

Intake in Overweight Adults," *Nutrition Journal* 12 (2013): 155, https://doi.org/10.1186/1475-2891-12-155.

15. "Top 25 Anthocyanin Rich Superfoods and Why You Should Eat Them," NaturalON: Natural Health News and Discoveries, accessed September 25, 2017, https://naturalon.com/top-25 -anthocyanin-rich-superfoods-and-why-you-should-eat-them/view -all/; see also In-Chul Lee, Dae Yong Kim, and Bu Young Choi, "Antioxidative Activity of Blueberry Leaf Extract Prevents High-Fat Diet-Induced Obesity in C57BL/6 Mice," *Journal of Cancer Prevention* 19, no. 3 (September 2014): 209–15, https://doi.org /10.15430/JCP.2014.19.3.209.

16. David Zinczenko, "7 Best Foods for Rapid Weight Loss," *Eat This, Not That!*, accessed June 12, 2017, http://www.eatthis .com/10-best-foods-rapid-weight-loss/.

17. K. Fujioka et al., "The Effects of Grapefruit on Weight and Insulin Resistance: Relationship to the Metabolic Syndrome," *Journal of Medicinal Food* 9, no. 1 (Spring 2006): 49–54, https://doi .org/10.1089/jmf.2006.9.49.

18. "22 Best Teas for Weight Loss," *Eat This, Not That!*, accessed June 10, 2017, http://www.eatthis.com/21-best-teas-for -weight-loss/.

19. Y. F. Li et al., "Tomato Juice Supplementation in Young Women Reduces Inflammatory Adipokine Levels Independently of Body Fat Reduction," *Nutrition* 31, no. 5 (May 2015): 691–6, https://doi.org/10.1016/j.nut.2014.11.008.

20. K. Couturier et al., "Cinnamon Improves Insulin Sensitivity and Alters the Body Composition in an Animal Model of the Metabolic Syndrome," *Archives of Biochemistry and Biophysics* 501,

no. 1 (September 1, 2010): 158–61, https://doi.org/10.1016/j.abb
.2010.05.032.

21. J. H. Kang et al., "Dietary Capsaicin Reduces Obesity-Induced Insulin Resistance and Hepatic Steatosis in Obese Mice Fed a High-Fat Diet," *Obesity* 18, no. 4 (April 2010): 780–7, https://doi.org/10.1038/oby.2009.301.

22. Caroline Praderio, "1 Daily Teaspoon of This Spice Could Help You Lose 3 Times as Much Body Fat," *Prevention*, March 23, 2015, https://www.prevention.com/weight-loss/weight-loss-tips/cumin-spice-weight-loss.

23. Muhammad S. Mansour et al., "Ginger Consumption Enhances the Thermic Effect of Food and Promotes Feelings of Satiety without Affecting Metabolic and Hormonal Parameters in Overweight Men: A Pilot Study," *Metabolism* 61, no. 10 (October 2012): 1347–52, http://dx.doi.org/10.1016/j.metabol.2012.03.016.

24. P. G. Bradford, "Curcumin and Obesity," *BioFactors* 39, no. 1 (January–February 2013): 78–87, https://doi.org/10.1002/biof.1074.

25. "The 55 Best Ways to Boost Your Metabolism," *Eat This, Not That!*

26. Kasandra Brabaw, "13 Herbs and Spices Scientifically Proven to Help You Lose Weight," *Prevention*, January 6, 2016, https://www.prevention.com/weight-loss/herbs-and-spices-for-weight-loss.

27. Bevin A. Clare, Richard S. Conroy, and Kevin Spelman, "The Diuretic Effect in Human Subjects of an Extract of *Taraxacum officinale* Folium Over a Single Day," *Journal of Alternative and Complementary Medicine* 15, no. 8 (August 2009): 929–34, https://doi.org/10.1089/acm.2008.0152.

28. Brabaw, "13 Herbs and Spices Scientifically Proven to Help You Lose Weight."

29. S. I. Krevdiyyeh and J. Usta, "Diuretic Effect and Mechanism of Action of Parsley," *Journal of Ethnopharmacology* 79, no. 3 (March 2002): 353–7, https://www.ncbi.nlm.nih.gov/pubmed /11849841.

30. "22 Best Teas for Weight Loss," *Eat This, Not That!*

31. "22 Best Teas for Weight Loss," *Eat This, Not That!*

32. "22 Best Teas for Weight Loss," *Eat This, Not That!*

33. "The 55 Best Ways to Boost Your Metabolism," *Eat This, Not That!*

34. "22 Best Teas for Weight Loss," *Eat This, Not That!*

35. Katherine Marko, "11 Amazing Health Benefits of Hawthorn Berries," Alternative Daily, November 15, 2016, http:// www.thealternativedaily.com/health-benefits-of-hawthorn-berries/; "Guide to Nautral Diuretics," Healthline, accessed December 11, 2017, https://www.healthline.com/health/natural-diuretics#2.

36. E. Jiménez-Ferrer et al., "Diuretic Effect of Compounds from Hibiscus Sabdariffa by Modulation of the Aldosterone Activity," *Planta Medica* 78, no. 18 (December 2012): 1893–8, https://doi.org/10.1055/s-0032-1327864.

37. J. Alarcón-Alonso et al., "Pharmacological Characterization of the Diuretic Effect of Hibiscus Sabdariffa Linn (Malvaceae) Extract," *Journal of Ethnopharmacology* 139, no. 3 (February 2012): 751–6, https://doi.org/10.1016/j.jep.2011.12.005.

38. Danilo Maciel Carneiro et al., "Randomized, Double-Blind Clinical Trial to Assess the Acute Diuretic Effect of *Equisetum*

arvense (Field Horsetail) in Healthy Volunteers," *Evidence-Based Complementary and Alternative Medicine* 2014 (2014), accessed July 4, 2017, http://dx.doi.org/10.1155/2014/760683.

39. "22 Best Teas for Weight Loss," *Eat This, Not That!*

40. "The 55 Best Ways to Boost Your Metabolism," *Eat This, Not That!*

41. "22 Best Teas for Weight Loss," *Eat This, Not That!*

42. "22 Best Teas for Weight Loss," *Eat This, Not That!*

43. "22 Best Teas for Weight Loss," *Eat This, Not That!*

44. "The 55 Best Ways to Boost Your Metabolism," *Eat This, Not That!*

45. Cynthia Sass, "Apple Cider Vinegar Helps Blood Sugar, Body Fat, Studies Say," *CNN Health+*, December 22, 2016, http://www.cnn.com/2016/12/22/health/apple-cider-vinegar-benefits/index.html; see also Tomoo Kondo et al., "Acetic Acid Upregulates the Expression of Genes for Fatty Acid Oxidation Enzymes in Liver to Suppress Body Fat Accumulation," *Journal of Agricultural and Food Chemistry* 57, no. 13 (2009): 5982–6, https://doi.org/0.1021/jf900470c.

46. Sass, "Apple Cider Vinegar Helps Blood Sugar, Body Fat, Studies Say"; see also T. Kondo et al., "Vinegar Intake Reduces Body Weight, Body Fat Mass, and Serum Triglyceride Levels in Obese Japanese Subjects," Bioscience, Biotechnology, and Biochemistry 73, no. 8 (August 2009): 1837–43, https://www.ncbi.nlm.nih.gov/pubmed/19661687.

47. Marc S. Micozzi, "Link Between Diet Soda and 'Diet-betes,'" OmniVista Health LLC, February 21, 2013, https://www.drmicozzi.com/link-between-diet-soda-and-diet-betes.

14. "Do Organic Fruits and Vegetables Taste Better Than Conventional Produce?," The Organic Center.

15. David Gutierrez, "Eating Organic Foods Reduces Pesticide Exposure by Nearly 90 Percent After Just One Week," *Natural News*, May 6, 2014, http://www.naturalnews.com/045006_organic _foods_pesticide_exposure_phthalates.html.

16. "Dirty Dozen: EWG's 2017 Shopper's Guide to Pesticides in Produce," Environmental Working Group, accessed March 31, 2017, https://www.ewg.org/foodnews/dirty_dozen_list.php.

17. "Clean Fifteen: EWG's 2017 Shopper's Guide to Pesticides in Produce," Environmental Working Group, accessed March 31, 2017, https://www.ewg.org/foodnews/clean_fifteen_list.php.

18. Simcha Weinstein, "Organic Produce From Mexico," Fresh Perspectives, March 19, 2013, http://blog.albertsorganics.com /?p=3098.

19. Weinstein, "Organic Produce From Mexico."

20. Weinstein, "Organic Produce From Mexico.

21. George L. Tritsch, quoted in "Potential Health Hazards of Food Irradiation: Verbatim Excerpts From Expert Testimony, U.S. Congressional Hearings into Food Irradiation," June 19, 1987, http://ccnr.org/food_irradiation.html.

22. Jeffrey Smith, "10 Reasons to Avoid GMOs," Institute for Responsible Technology, August 25, 2011, http://responsible technology.org/10-reasons-to-avoid-gmos/.

23. Jeffrey M. Smith, "Articles About Health Risks by Jeffrey Smith," Institute for Responsible Technology, accessed June 20, 2017, http://responsibletechnology.org/gmo-education/articles -about-health-risks-by-jeffrey.

24. Maria Rodale and Alberto Gonzalez, "12 Reasons to Avoid GMOS," *HuffPost: The Blog*, January 31, 2012, http://www.huffingtonpost.com/maria-rodale/12-reasons-to-avoid-gmos_b_1243723.html.

25. David Derbyshire, "Fears Grow as Study Shows Genetically Modified Crops 'Can Cause Liver and Kidney Damage,'" *Daily Mail*, January 21, 2010, http://www.dailymail.co.uk/news/article-1244824/Fears-grow-study-shows-genetically-modified-crops-cause-liver-kidney-damage.html.

26. Joël Spiroux de Vendômois et al., "A Comparison of the Effects of Three GM Corn Varieties on Mammalian Health," *International Journal of Biological Sciences* 5, no. 7 (2009): 706–26, https://doi.org/10.7150/ijbs.5.706.

27. Smith, "10 Reasons to Avoid GMOs."

28. Smith, "10 Reasons to Avoid GMOs."

29. James E. McWilliams, "The Green Monster," Slate.com, January 28, 2009, accessed February 8, 2010, http://www.slate.com/id/2209168/pagenum/all/.

CHAPTER 5 | CHOOSING YOUR BEST MOVES

1. Ashley Oerman, "7 Reasons to Try High-Intensity Interval Training," *Women's Health*, August 14, 2014, https://www.womenshealthmag.com/fitness/high-intensity-interval-training.

2. Stephen H. Boutcher, "High-Intensity Intermittent Exercise and Fat Loss," *Journal of Obesity* 2011 (2011): 868305, https://doi.org/10.1155/2011/868305.

3. Glenn Riseley, "19 Reasons Why Cycling Is the Best Exercise," *HuffPost*, August 14, 2015, http://www.huffingtonpost.com

/glenn-riseley/19-reasons-why-cycling-is-the-best-exercise_b_7974474.html.

4. Alyssa Shaffer, "Walk Off 5 Times More Belly Fat," *Prevention*, November 3, 2011, https://www.prevention.com/fitness/fitness-tips/lose-your-belly-fat-8-week-walking-workout.

5. A. Bhattacharya et al., "Body Acceleration Distribution and O2 Uptake in Humans during Running and Jumping," *Journal of Applied Physiology* 49, no. 5 (November 1, 1980): 881–7, http://jap.physiology.org/content/49/5/881.

6. Jaliyah Dinard, "15 Yoga Poses You Should Be Doing Everyday," Spoon University Inc., June 4, 2016, https://spoonuniversity.com/lifestyle/15-yoga-poses-everyday.

7. Christian Nordqvist, "Metabolism: Myths and Facts," *Medical News Today*, last updated July 18, 2017, https://www.medicalnewstoday.com/articles/8871.php; see also "Exercise Reverses Unhealthy Effects of Inactivity," ScienceDaily, June 3, 2006, https://www.sciencedaily.com/releases/2006/06/060603091830.htm.

CHAPTER 6 | WHEN WEIGHT LOSS PLATEAUS HAPPEN TO GOOD PEOPLE

1. "I Would Spend 55 Minutes Defining the Problem and Then Five Minutes Solving It," Quote Investigator, accessed June 2, 2017, http://quoteinvestigator.com/2014/05/22/solve/.

2. AZ Quotes, Charlotte Gerson, accessed June 2, 2017, http://www.azquotes.com/quote/912925.

3. Josh Axe, "9 Ways to Boost Glutathione," DrAxe.com, accessed June 13, 2017, https://draxe.com/glutathione/; see also Nicole Cutler, "8 Great Foods for Detoxing the Liver,"

Liversupport.com, September 30, 2014, http://www.liversupport
.com/8-great-foods-for-detoxing-the-liver/.

4.   Cutler, "8 Great Foods for Detoxing the Liver."

5.   Cutler, "8 Great Foods for Detoxing the Liver."

6.   "What Is Glucose?," WebMD, accessed June 17, 2017,
http://www.webmd.com/diabetes/glucose-diabetes#1.

7.   P. D. Tsitouras et al., "High Omega-3 Fat Intake Improves
Insulin Sensitivity and Reduces CRP and IL6, but Does Not
Affect Other Endocrine Axes in Healthy Older Adults," *Hormone
and Metabolic Research* 40, no. 3 (March 2008): 199–205, https://
doi.org/10.1055/s-2008-1046759.

8.   E. Donga et al. "A Single Night of Partial Sleep Deprivation Induces Insulin Resistance in Multiple Metabolic Pathways in
Healthy Subjects," *Journal of Clinical Endocrinology and Metabolism*
95, no. 6 (June 2010): 2963–8, https://doi.org/10.1210/jc.2009
-2430.

9.   "What Is Gestational Diabetes?," American Diabetes Association, last updated November 21, 2016, http://www.diabetes.org
/diabetes-basics/gestational/what-is-gestational-diabetes.html.

10.   Mayo Clinic Staff, "Metabolic Syndrome," accessed June 17,
2017, http://www.mayoclinic.org/diseases-conditions/metabolic
-syndrome/home/ovc-20197517.

11.   "Artificial Sweeteners Linked to Weight Gain," American
Psychological Association, accessed June 23, 2017, https://news
.uns.purdue.edu/x/2008a/080211SwithersAPA.html; see also S. E.
Swithers and T. L. Davidson, "A Role for Sweet Taste: Calorie
Predictive Relations in Energy Regulation by Rats," *Behavioral*

Neuroscience 122, no. 1 (February 2008): 161–73, https://doi.org /10.1037/0735-7044.122.1.161.

12. Kate S. Collison et al., "Gender Dimorphism in Aspartame-Induced Impairment of Spatial Cognition and Insulin Sensitivity," *PLOS One* 7, no. 4 (April 3, 2012): e31570, https://doi.org/10.1371 /journal.pone.0031570.

13. Fernando de Matos Feijó et al., "Saccharin and Aspartame, Compared with Sucrose, Induce Greater Weight Gain in Adult Wistar Rats, at Similar Total Caloric Intake Levels," *Appetite* 60 (January 1, 2013): 203–7, https://doi.org/10.1016/j.appet.2012 .10.009.

14. Benyagoub Mohamed et al., "Splenda Alters Gut Microflora and Increases Intestinal P-Glycoprotein and Cytochrome P-450 in Male Rats," *Journal of Toxicology and Environmental Health* 71 (February 2008): 1415–29, https://doi.org /10.1080/15287390802328630.

15. "Gender and Stress," American Psychological Association, accessed June 29, 2017, http://www.apa.org/news/press/releases /stress/2010/gender-stress.aspx.

16. "Gender and Stress," American Psychological Association.

17. "Sleep Deprivation Linked to Weight Gain," Medscape Conference Coverage, based on selected sessions at the American Thoracic Society 2006 International Conference, May 24, 2006, https://www.medscape.com/viewarticle/533105.

18. "Sleep Deprivation Linked to Weight Gain," Medscape Conference Coverage.

19. Mark Hyman, "How Hidden Food Sensitivities Make You Fat," Dr.Hyman.com, accessed July 7, 2017, http://drhyman.com/blog/2012/02/22/how-hidden-food-sensitivities-make-you-fat/.

20. Josh Axe, "Are You Eating a High-Fiber Diet?," Dr.Axe.com, accessed July 8, 2017, https://draxe.com/high-fiber-diet/.

21. "Gut Microbiota Info: Everything You Always Wanted to Know About the Gut Microbiota...," Gut Microbiota for Health, accessed July 9, 2017, http://www.gutmicrobiotaforhealth.com/en/about-gut-microbiota-info/.

22. Brenda Watson, renowned authority in digestive health, in communication with the author.

23. Gudmundur Bergsson et al., "In Vitro Killing of Candida albicans by Fatty Acids and Monoglycerides," *Antimicrobial Agents and Chemotherapy* 45, no. 11 (November 2001): 3209–12, https://doi.org/10.1128/AAC.45.11.3209-3212.2001.

CHAPTER 7 | SIPPING SKINNY MENU PLANS

1. Carolyn M. Gallagher and Jaymie R. Meliker, "Mercury and Thyroid Autoantibodies in U.S. Women, NHANES 2007–2008," *Environment International* 40 (April 2012): 39–43, https://doi.org/10.1016/j.envint.2011.11.014.

2. "José N. Harris Quotes," GoodReads, accessed September 27, 2017, https://www.goodreads.com/quotes/415120-to-get-something-you-never-had-you-have-to-do.

CHAPTER 8 | SIPPING SKINNY RECIPES

1.   Jack Challoner, "How Soup Can Help You Lose Weight," *BBC News Magazine*, last updated May 26, 2009, http://news.bbc .co.uk/2/hi/uk_news/magazine/8068733.stm.